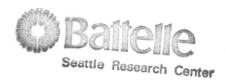

Battelle
Seattle Research Center

After Barney Clark

REFLECTIONS ON THE UTAH ARTIFICIAL HEART PROGRAM

Proceedings of a conference held at Alta, Utah, 13–15 October 1983, and cosponsored by the University of Utah and The University of Texas Health Science Center at Houston

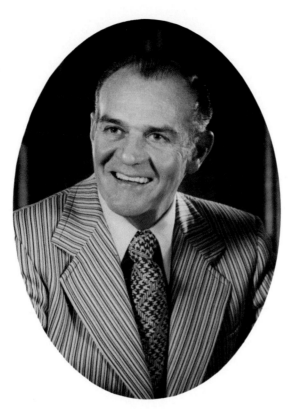

All in all, it's been a pleasure to be able to help people.
BARNEY B. CLARK, D.D.S. (1921–1983)

After Barney Clark

REFLECTIONS ON THE
UTAH ARTIFICIAL HEART
PROGRAM

Edited by
Margery W. Shaw

 UNIVERSITY OF TEXAS PRESS, AUSTIN

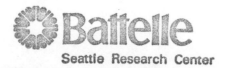

Seattle Research Center

LIBRARY OF CONGRESS CATALOGING IN PUBLICATION DATA
Main entry under title:
After Barney Clark.
    Proceedings of a conference held Oct. 13–15, 1983, in
Alta, Utah, and sponsored by the University of Utah and
the University of Texas Health Science Center at Houston.
    Includes bibliographical references and index.
    1. Heart, Artificial—Congresses.   2. Clark, Barney B.,
1921–1983.   3. Heart—Surgery—Complications and sequelae
—Congresses.   I. Shaw, Margery W., 1923–
II. University of Utah.   III. University of Texas Health
Science Center at Houston.   [DNLM: 1. Clark, Barney B.,
1921–1983.   2. Heart, Artificial—congresses.
WG169.5 A258   1983]
RD598.A38   1984   362.1'97412   84-10394
ISBN 0-292-70376-7

Contents

Preface

Barney B. Clark, a Seattle dentist, arrived for surgery at the University of Utah Medical Center by helicopter from the airport around 5:00 P.M. on Monday, 29 November 1982. Several months previously he had been evaluated by Dr. Jeffrey Anderson, a cardiologist at the University of Utah Medical Center, who had referred him to Dr. William DeVries, a thoracic surgeon, as a possible candidate for an artificial heart implant. At that time Dr. DeVries had discussed the procedure, the risks, and the potential benefits of implanting an artificial heart. They had visited the laboratories where the pump was manufactured and the animal barn where they observed calves and sheep with heart implants. Dr. Clark had asked many questions concerning the reliability (and failures) of the artificial heart and the cause of death of the animals who had undergone implantation. Dr. DeVries gave Dr. Clark a copy of the informed consent form (Appendix A), which had been approved by the University of Utah Institutional Review Board for Research with Human Subjects (IRB) and the federal Food and Drug Administration. After their meeting, Dr. Clark returned to Seattle and discussed the operation with family and friends and also with his Seattle cardiologist, Dr. Terence Block. Dr. Clark concluded that he alone would decide if and when he would consent to the implant procedure, regardless of the advice of others.

During the weeks between his meeting with Dr. DeVries and his arrival at the Utah medical center, Dr. Clark's cardiac status had continued to deteriorate until he was bedridden, required oxygen supplementation, and had persistent dyspnea, even at rest. He called Dr. DeVries and requested surgery.

Dr. Clark's diagnosis on admission was idiopathic cardiomyopathy with Class IV congestive heart failure. His cardiac output was one liter per minute (normal range, six to seven liters per minute), and he had ascites and peripheral edema that were not responding well to diuretics. He was considered to be moribund.

Dr. Clark was interviewed on Tuesday, 30 November, by six members of a special heart subcommittee of the IRB who unanimously approved him as a candidate for implantation. The eleven-page consent form was thoroughly reviewed with him by Dr. De-Vries and Ross Woolley, Ph.D. At 8:30 P.M. on 29 November he signed the informed consent document (see Appendix A). He signed the form again at 9:52 P.M. on 30 November.

Surgery was scheduled for the morning of 2 December; however, Dr. Clark's condition worsened on 1 December, and it was feared that he might not survive through the night. He was wheeled into the surgical suite at 11:00 P.M. Wednesday, 1 December, and the operation ended at 7:05 A.M. on Thursday, 2 December. He was placed in the intensive care unit (ICU) in stable but serious condition.

His immediate postoperative course was stormy. Crepitation was noted in the chest wall, and surgery was required to repair several air leaks from ruptured alveoli (air sacs in the lungs) on 4 December. On 7 December, his sixth postoperative day, he suffered generalized and focal seizures of undetermined origin, but these were thought to be caused by a metabolic imbalance. During the next three weeks his mental state was confused but gradually improved with intervening periods of lucidity.

On 14 December a sudden drop in blood pressure because of a broken valve required surgery to replace the left ventricle of the artificial heart. A stress fracture on the housing of the mitral valve, which had been thought to be an extremely unlikely event, caused the complication. Because of anticoagulant medication to prevent blood clots, Dr. Clark suffered severe nosebleeds in early January, requiring nose packs and eventual surgery on 18 January 1983.

On 14 February Dr. Clark's condition was upgraded from serious to fair, and he was moved from the surgical ICU to a private room, but he returned to the ICU the next day because of his need for a respirator. On 24 February he was again returned to a private room where his condition gradually improved.

During January and February he gained increasing strength by passive and active exercises. He also made visits to other parts of the hospital in his wheelchair and had frequent visitors at his bedside. On 1 March he was interviewed by Dr. DeVries, and the session was videotaped. Preparations were under way for transfer to a residence in Salt Lake City where his cardiac monitoring system would be networked to a university hospital computer and video screen.

On 3 March he suffered a temporary setback from aspiration pneumonia, which cleared with antibiotic therapy. On 21 March his clinical course deteriorated again with reduced renal function and fever. Two days later, on 23 March at 10:02 P.M., he died of circulatory collapse because of multiorgan system failure.

Dr. Clark was the first person to live with an artificial heart that was implanted as a permanent, rather than a temporary, replacement for his own heart. He survived 112 days, and the artificial heart had sustained Dr. Clark with 12,912,499 beats.

In early 1983 I had the opportunity to visit the University of Utah medical school and to meet most of the participants in the drama that was then unfolding. I became aware of the many practical day-to-day decisions being made by the Utah heart team and the ethical, social, economic, and political overtones in these decisions. During discussions with university administrator Dr. Chase N. Peterson a conference was planned to bring together national experts to carry on further dialogue with the local participants in the artificial heart program. We hoped for an open and frank exchange. We also felt it would be important to communicate our deliberations to the general public.

The conference was held at Alta, Utah, 13–15 October 1983. This book contains the papers that were presented and summaries of audience discussions at that meeting. (There is no summary of the Part Three papers, which were presented following a banquet.) Appendix A contains a copy of the informal consent form signed by Barney Clark, and Appendix B lists the publications of the chief surgeon, William C. DeVries.

Approximately thirty people from the University of Utah attended in addition to the contributors of this volume. We had a rare opportunity for frank discussions with the Utah group, giving us a unique inside look at this historical event that captured the attention of the nation and the world. Our readers may now share in this intimate colloquy.

I gratefully acknowledge the permission granted by Free Press, a division of Macmillan, to reprint an excerpt from chapter 6 of *The Silent World of Doctor and Patient* by Jay Katz (1984). I also thank Marilyn Howard, whose efficiency in making the local arrangements for the conference helped make the meeting an enjoyable experience. A special debt of gratitude is owed to Betty Goodrum, who cheerfully typed the entire manuscript and assisted in editing and indexing.

PART ONE

Ethical Perspectives

Setting the Tone of the Conference

MARGERY W. SHAW

We, as human beings, are planners, designers, builders, and achievers. We tinker, explore, invent, and create. This is part of our genetic heritage. We are the survivors of the natural selection process of human biological evolution. Our recent brain development has propelled us into a cultural evolution that has outstripped the capacities of our physical selves. Our vital organs break down, but our brains compel us to fix them, to renovate them, and to replace them. Technology and innovation are part of our inner drives. It should come as no surprise to anyone that, sooner or later, an artificial heart would be implanted in the chest of one of our fellow human beings.

But we are also subject to other needs and drives. We dream, believe, hope, aspire, and trust. We also deny, doubt, and despair. These struggles create conflicts. We need to rest, reflect, and recuperate, while at the same time, we are propelled to achieve and progress and succeed.

This conference brings us together to explore our human struggles as we discuss and evaluate the artificial heart implant program. The Utah heart team, after fifteen years of research and development and more than four hundred animal experiments, took a brave new step in December 1982. The team has given us a unique challenge to reflect on that achievement that has excited a world of people.

The creation of the artificial is a natural instinct. If the artificial heart is "unnatural," it can only be so in the sense that all of medicine is. Joseph Fletcher said, "To oppose technology is self-hatred."[1] Joshua Lederberg, once addressing those who would stop the learning process, said, "The suppression of knowledge appears to me unthinkable, not only on ideological but on merely logical grounds. How can the ignorant know what they should not know?"[2]

Perhaps Lewis Thomas said it best of all in his "Notes of a Biology Watcher":

Is there something fundamentally unnatural, or intrinsically wrong, or hazardous for the species, in the ambition that drives us all to reach a comprehensive understanding of nature, including ourselves? I cannot believe it. It would seem to me a more unnatural thing, and more of an offense against nature, for us to come on the scene endowed as we are with curiosity, and naturally talented as we are for the asking of clear questions, and then for us to do nothing about it, or worse, to try to suppress the questions. This is the great danger of our species, to try to pretend that we are another kind of animal . . . and that the human mind can rise above its ignorance by simply asserting there are things it has no need to know. This, to my way of thinking, is the real hubris, and it carries danger for us all.[3]

It is easy to establish a rationale—our innate curiosity and inventiveness—for traversing the road of progress in the development of a man-made implantable heart device that replaces Nature's own. But the road ahead of us has obstacles that should be addressed in order to justify continuation of the project. We need to consider the selection of patients, the just allocation of a scarce resource, the economic costs, and other sociological and ethical issues. That is why we have gathered together for these three days. We acknowledge the graciousness of our hosts at Utah who have invited us here to explore these issues with them in a constructive, but critical way.

NOTES

1. J. Fletcher, *Humanhood: Essays in Biomedical Ethics* (Buffalo, N.Y.: Prometheus Books, 1979), p. 17.

2. J. Lederberg, "Orthobiosis, the Perfection of Man," in *The Place of Values in a World of Facts*, ed. A. Tiselius and S. Nilsson, p. 174 (New York: John Wiley & Sons, 1971).

3. L. Thomas, "Notes of a Biology Watcher," *New England Journal of Medicine* 296 (10 February 1977): 328.

The Selection of Patients

ALBERT R. JONSEN

Dr. Chase Peterson, gracious host of the conference, is reported as having once said that Dr. Barney Clark was like Columbus. The analogy is, in part, apt. Dr. Clark had the willingness to venture into the unknown and the bravery to face its dangers. The analogy is also, in part, unsuitable. Columbus was not only a bold adventurer but—if we heed his historian, Admiral Samuel Eliot Morrison—he was one of the most skilled navigators of his time. He dreamed, but he could also plot a course toward the horizon better than any other sailor. Dr. Clark was not like Columbus, the skilled planner and captain of a voyage but was rather the object of planning, the fragile caravel that was sailed rather than the sailor. The analogy mimics history in another way. Within two decades of Columbus's journey, his discoveries had become the scene of a vivid moral drama. The Americas were the arena of a bitter crisis of justice and fairness: To whom should these lands belong? Were its indigenous peoples the entitled rulers or unwilling victims? Intellectual opinion in Europe was riven, and despite the contrary opinions of learned theologians, the monstrous injustices of the European conquest of the Americas bloodied the sixteenth century.

What has this to do with the cardiac implant? If Dr. Clark is a Columbus, his brave venture should be seen as the prelude to a crisis of justice and fairness. Who can lay claim to the fragile caravel in which Barney Clark's life rode for 112 days? How is the society of discoverers to parcel out the benefit of life launched in the stormy days of December 1982? We ought not only to remember Barney Clark as the brave and lonely navigator in uncharted seas but also as the precursor of a unique social crisis. What he volunteered to undergo was the exploratory voyage opening territories on which new claimants will seize shores and many others will be dispossessed. The metaphor of Columbus is the metaphor for the ethical problem of selection of subjects.

At risk of exhausting my metaphor, I point out that voyages of discovery pose two problems: how to get to where one hopes to get and what to do with the new lands once arrived. In medicine, the two phases are the experimental phase, the problem of getting there, and the therapeutic phase, the best use of what one has got. Each of these phases is quite different in technical, psychological, and ethical ways. From the ethical viewpoint, the experimental phase is dominated by the utilitarian principle: so act as to produce the greatest good for the greatest number. (For my colleagues who are not tainted by the technical language of philosophy, "utilitarian" is not a pejorative term meaning exploitive, nor the economist's measure of production; it is a philosophical term that identifies action as moral exclusively in terms of the benefits effected by that action.) Although the ethics of biomedical research has hedged around the principle of utility with the principle of respect for autonomy, which demands the informed consent of research participants, the moral justification for research itself remains the ultimate benefits of new knowledge and new therapeutics. Risks are thereby morally permitted that would not otherwise be, just as a voyage of discovery may tolerate greater dangers than subsequent commercial trips.

The application of the principle of utility not only justifies risks in view of future benefits, it also suggests that steps be taken to arrive most efficiently at the goal. Thus, among the requisites of good research, from both the technical and the ethical viewpoint, is the selection of subjects "ideal" to yield the information sought. Choice of subjects less than ideal can contaminate the research and so fail to produce the benefits of new knowledge and therapies. Again, an ethical limit is placed on the utilitarian rule: it is the classical moral maxim of medicine—"Do no harm."

The utilitarian principle, the principle of autonomy, and the principle of—oh, miserable word—nonmaleficence all appear in three episodes of the history of experimentation of human subjects. The earliest remark about this subject comes from the third-century Roman physician Celsus, who approved of the vivisection of criminals for research with the words, "It is not cruel to inflict on a few criminals, sufferings which may benefit multitudes of innocent persons throughout the ages." Sixteen centuries later, Claude Bernard, father of experimental medicine, stated, "The principle of medical morality consists in never performing on man an experiment which might be harmful to him to any extent, though the result might be highly advantageous to science and to the health of others." In the first decade of our century, the incomparable Sir William Osler justified the yellow fever experiments of Walter Reed by noting that although they exposed the subjects to risk of death, the subjects had freely volunteered themselves for this known risk. Thus, utility, nonmaleficence, and autonomy govern the experimental phase. They govern, of course, in theory; for in practice they are not always easily compatible. One of them, and it is usually the primary principle of utility, must yield to the others. In the case of selection of patients for artificial heart implant, the incompatibility of these ethical principles is obvious and agonizing.

The recipient of the yet imperfect device with still uncertain consequences should be "ideal" from the utilitarian viewpoint: being that sort of research subject from whom best and maximum information can be gained, information leading to a perfected device with certain consequences. At the same time, the experiment involves one lethal step, the removal of that recipient's own heart. This incurs not the risk of death, as do many other experiments, but the certainty of death, unless the function of the original heart is not almost immediately replaced. The only parallel I know in modern medicine is bone marrow transplantation in which hematopoiesis must be radically suppressed before transplant. Thus, initiation of the experiment itself will, to paraphrase Bernard, without doubt do harm to a great extent. It will kill the recipient. Like the vivisection mentioned by Celsus, it removes an organ necessary for life. We cannot justify this, as Celsus did, by reference to the greater good of the greater number.

In order to hedge the utilitarian principle, we seek out a person who will be able to give free consent, as Osler advised. The challenge of free and informed consent is enormous in this situation. Will you accept certainty of death or the high risk of death in order to provide us with new information? This is a question few but the most heroic and altruistic would answer in the affirmative. So we go not to these but to the most vulnerable: to a person almost dead and with no hope other than this remote one offered by the imperfect device with the uncertain consequences. For the free consent of such a person we must remedy, not only the patient's ignorance about pathophysiology, physics, and prognosis—a relatively simple task—but also the coercions of fear and hope—a much more difficult and unlikely one. Again, when we do find such mortally ill persons who can and will consent as freely and fully as possible—and it appears that Dr. Clark was such a person—we have compromised the utilitarian principle under which the research was initiated. We have a subject less than ideal for the purpose of the most and best information.

Faced with this paradox, the temptation is to turn the experiment into a purported therapy. The procedure is done, it is said and perhaps believed, in order to save the recipient's life, to give again the health now ruined by a pathologically incompetent heart. The frank and, in itself, moral principle of utility is buried beneath the weight of the principle of beneficence focused on this recipient, not on future generations of heart patients. Possibly, we cannot do otherwise psychologically. We have selected a suffering human being who is willing to do us a great favor through his continued suffering. Can we, his fellow humans, do otherwise than hope that the success of this experiment will include his well-being? Yet, in so doing, the impression is created that a therapy has been discovered. The imperfections and the uncertainties are muted; the possibilities of hope, cure, and health are heralded. Even the recipient himself is pictured as returning to health; the desperately ill man now smiles, even walks. Even the most discreet physicians and most circumspect scientists and the most cautious publicists cannot counter the therapeutic impression. They themselves quite naturally share it. They are not cold and impartial observers. Yet, it is important to note that this shift in the psychology and perception of the experimental phase has implications for the ethics of patient selection.

Once the voyage of discovery has pitched on a previously unknown territory, the problem of possession and distribution appears. This, in medical care, is the therapeutic phase. Traditionally, the ethics of this phase has not reflected the problems of possession and distribution; the ethics of therapy has been governed by the principle expressed in lapidary form in the Hippocratic literature: to help or at least to do no harm. No footnote tells us to whom help is due. It has always been assumed that help is due to those sufferers who come for care. The ethical fulcrum of all actions in the therapeutic phase is the sufferer, not society at large. All duties center on the benefits that medical intervention can bring to the individual seeking help. The utilitarian principle, at least in its global formulation, cedes to the principle of beneficence and nonmaleficence. Now, however, a new problem appears.

Many technological interventions are scarce and costly; they have been developed by society's contributions and have consequences of importance for the society as a whole. This is now recognized more forthrightly by physicians, scientists, and policymakers than in the past. The following question now arises: should the utilitarian principle, usually assiduously banished from therapeutics, be reintroduced? If so, what weight or priority should it have in ethical decisions in clinical medicine? The question applies to the selection of patients. Should the choice of those who will be given a therapeutic benefit usually made in view of the ethical principle of beneficence and nonmaleficence toward an individual sufferer, be made, instead, in view of a principle of social utility? Since the scarce and costly resource cannot come to all in need, should it come to those in need whose personal benefit represents the highest and best use for society? We face a classical ethical problem long familiar to political and economic life but unfamiliar to medicine—the problem of justice.

The ethicists now ask how, that is, in accord with what principles, can a therapy be distributed fairly and justly. Some have suggested that fairness can be served only by random selection methods such as lotteries. Critics have responded that the results of a lottery would bestow precious resources on some persons who have done poorly by society and little deserve its bounty. This, they say, also violates justice. Ethicists have suggested queuing as a method of serving justice. Critics have responded that queuing favors the privileged who have means of arriving early and that it cannot take account of the variable course of clinical illness. Finally, some ethicists have frankly espoused a utilitarian approach: the choice of most suitable patients, in terms of their social productivity and promise, is justified because society is entitled to a return on its investment.

We are only on the verge of the debate about the ethical use of scarce and costly technology. We encountered the problem most starkly with the advent of renal dialysis and kidney transplants in the 1960s. A flurry of debate about the ethics of selection was stirred up. It subsided when the End Stage Renal Disease Amendments were funded. It is stirring again as the cost of the ESRD program becomes controversial. We must not allow the ethical analysis of this problem to rise and fall with dramatic discoveries. We must persist in a careful consideration of a problem of selection posed by new technologies. We should, however, be more prescient of the claims that will be made on newly discovered therapies than was Columbus about the claims to be laid on newly discovered lands. A heart implant in some future Barney Clark may be a therapeutic triumph, but it will immediately be not merely the benefit enjoyed by that fortunate person but the property on which thousands of unfortunates will lay claim. A question our society seems unwilling to ask itself is whether a technology should be withheld from application unless and until it can be determined clearly how it can be distributed in a way that does not violate ethical principles of justice. On the optimistic side, this technology is destined to provide a new world for those to be exiled from life.

I have in these remarks stated two conundrums. First, the experimental phase of implants, which can be rightly governed by the utilitarian principle, encounters obstacles set by the ethics of therapeutics. Choice of ideal research subjects is restricted by the imperatives to help or do no harm, imperatives that, at the experimental phase, may be almost impossible to respect and at the same time fulfill the utilitarian imperative of research. Second, as the implant becomes, or appears to become, a genuine therapy, we seem compelled to replace the beneficence principle that has commanded unwavering fidelity to the patient by the utilitarian principle that commands a cost-benefit attention to the social good.

I say these are conundrums, that is, problems for which there seems no satisfactory solution, yet most serious ethical problems appear to be conundrums at some point in their history. For a few of them, long reflection and experience leads to the conclusion that we have a genuine paradox: two equally imperative principles in direct conflict. For most, however, experience and reflection show ways to resolve the issue. This resolution, however, will elude us if we fail to recognize the tension, the uneasy fit of the ethics of research and therapy. This calls for two honest admissions: First, the next series of implants will be experiments with utilitarian purpose, not therapeutic benefits for sufferers. Second, the stage of therapeutic benefit, should it ever be reached, will impose on therapy the unfamiliar demands of social utility.

The ethics of patient selection, in both experimental and therapeutic phases of the artificial heart, is a complex issue. But even before we plunge into its complexity, we need the simple honesty of those two admissions. Barney Clark, despite his bravery, was not Columbus. You scientists and surgeons are the Columbuses, and you face a similar moral question: when is it morally right, given the uncertainties and the dangers, to set out on the voyage, and what is to be done once the voyage brings back news of a landfall on a highly desirable shore?

Patient Autonomy and the Process of Informed Consent

JAY KATZ

Physicians are well trained to attend caringly to patients' physical needs. Their education has not prepared them to attend caringly to patients' decision-making needs. Reconciling respect for self-determination with respect for patients' adult and childlike longings is a difficult undertaking. How to achieve such a reconciliation through conversation requires intensive study. In this chapter I shall apply some of the lessons to be learned from the theoretical explorations of the concept of psychological autonomy and the principle of self-determination to clinical situations.

The encounters of Louis Washkansky and Philip Blaiberg—the first and second persons to receive heart transplants—with their surgeon Christiaan Barnard, illustrate the importance of the internal component of self-determination (thinking about choices) for protecting patients' and doctors' psychological autonomy. These clinical examples are dramatic because of the extraordinary nature of the intervention itself, but they are not atypical. The failure to bring significant factors that affect physicians' and patients' choices to self-awareness and to the awareness of the other is common to everyday interactions between physicians and patients. I chose these examples because of the rare availability of reminiscences about the same event by both physician and patient.

THE FIRST TWO HEART TRANSPLANT PATIENTS

I shall begin with Blaiberg's description of his first meeting with Barnard the day after his admission to the hospital:

. . . I was lying in bed with eyes closed, feeling drowsy and thoroughly miserable when I sensed someone at the head of my bed. I opened my eyes and saw a man. He was tall, young, good-looking with features that reminded me a lot of General Jan Christian Smuts in his later years. His hands were beautiful; the hands of the born surgeon.

"Don't you know me?" he asked.

"No," I said with little interest, "I don't."

"I'm Professor Chris Barnard," he said.

"I'm sorry, Professor," I replied, "but I didn't recognize you. I have never seen you in person, and you look so different from your photographs in the Press."

He spoke earnestly. "Dr. Blaiberg, how do you feel about the prospect of a heart transplant operation? You probably know, don't you, that I am prepared to do you next?"

"The sooner the better," I said fervently, "and I promise you my full cooperation at all times."

Though our conversation was brief and he stayed only a few minutes, I was immediately impressed with the stature of the man and his air of buoyant optimism. He inspired me with the greatest confidence, an invaluable asset in the relations between a surgeon and his patient.

I felt somewhat better. Here was a man to whom I would willingly entrust my life. I came to know him well in the weeks and months that followed. He is a vital, determined, somewhat mercurial, personality, utterly dedicated to his profession.[1]

A few days later, the morning after Washkansky had died, news that had been kept from Blaiberg, Barnard came to see him again. As Blaiberg remembered it,

[Barnard] was haggard and drawn as though he had not slept all night. He no longer resembled the handsome Smuts, to whom I had compared him, but more a martyred Christ. I felt a twinge of pity for him when I noticed the pain in his face and eyes. Something, I was sure, had happened to dampen the gaiety and boundless optimism I had seen before.

*   *   *   *

Professor Barnard spoke in low tones. "I feel like a pilot who has just crashed," he said. "Now I want you, Dr. Blaiberg, to help me by taking up another plane as soon as possible to get back my confidence."

Still I did not know what he was driving at. "Professor," I said, puzzled, "why are you telling me this? You know I am prepared to undergo a heart transplant operation at any time you wish."

"But don't you know that Louis Washkansky is dead?" he asked. "He died this morning, of pneumonia."

. . . Now I knew the reason for his distress and agitation.

"Professor Barnard," I said at once, "I want to go through with it now more than ever—not only for my sake but for you and your team who put so much into your effort to save Louis Washkansky."

Blaiberg's description of his initial meeting with Barnard vividly depicts the preemptory emergence of infantile modes of behavior in patients that at least for a while can drown out adult reasoning and reflection. Barnard instantaneously became in Blaiberg's mind an omnipotent parent and hero. He was no longer only a surgeon who would do his level best to prolong life. He also had become a representative of many of the powerful persons Blaiberg had encountered in his life. For example, Barnard became General Smuts, under whom Blaiberg had served and whom he admired greatly. From the first moment he had laid his eyes on Barnard, Blaiberg idealized him. Unquestioning, he placed himself in "the [beautiful] hands of the born surgeon . . . utterly dedicated to his profession," and willingly entrusted his life to him.

In their second meeting, Barnard also became Christ, the powerful protector. Yet, he was the "martyred Christ," who had given His life for the sake of mankind. But it was Blaiberg, not Barnard, who was perhaps prepared to be a martyr for the sake of mankind. Is it not possible that when Blaiberg "noticed the pain in [Barnard's] face and eyes," he unconsciously identified with him, projected his own "distress and agitation" onto Barnard, made him the martyred Christ, and confused his own identity with that of his surgeon? Recall that Blaiberg now wanted to go through with the operation not only for his own sake but for the sake of Barnard and his team as well. If Barnard had suspected that Blaiberg could react in some such fashion, he might have first inquired about how Blaiberg viewed him, and then talked with him about his human limitations as a surgeon, about the limitations of his craft, and, in this instance, about his own uncertainties of providing Blaiberg with the relief that he expected from this novel operation. As a result of such conversations, Blaiberg might eventually have recognized his confusion of Barnard with his life-giving parents, as well as with the real and storybook heroes of his past, and, in turn, placed his surgeon in better perspective.

Patients, particularly those in the throes of serious illness, characteristically become confused about past and present. Barnard's extensive clinical experience must have made him aware of this phenomenon. That he did not attend to it in this instance is another matter. Yet, such inattentiveness raises questions about his responsibilities to recognize such a common reaction, and attempt, through sustained conversations, to moderate Blaiberg's infantile fantasies about him and about the success of the operation. The responsibility for engaging in such conversations cannot be assigned to Blaiberg, it rests with his doctor.

It is most likely, however, that any thoughts Barnard might have entertained of subjecting his patient's magical expectations to reflection and critical appraisal were obliterated by his self-interested eagerness to perform another transplant on a suitable patient as soon as possible. His zeal to forge ahead conflicted with the many doubts Barnard must have entertained about the promise of a procedure never before performed on man. Such disquieting doubts generally tend to be suppressed rather than confronted. They seem to disturb "the courage, grit, or guts" that transplant surgeons have emphasized as being so essential to their work.[2] Yet, as long as such suppressions are deemed essential to effectiveness, they invariably will lead to silence about important matters that deserve discussion.

Thus, another question arises: Was it Barnard's responsibility to become aware of the fact that his own interests might conflict with those of his patient? If he had regarded it as his responsibility, the conflicts would have emerged more readily in conversations with Blaiberg. With some encouragement, Blaiberg might have raised a number of perplexing and disturbing questions about the operation. Since Barnard did not wish to, or could not, own up to his doubts and conflicts, he surely was not prepared to evoke them in his patient. Instead, he all too quickly said, "[G]ood. I'll come again soon," and took his leave.[3]

Some time earlier Barnard had similarly avoided conversation with Washkansky's wife, Ann. When she had asked, "What chances do you give him?" he had responded without hesitation or further explanation, "An 80 percent chance." This response was utterly meaningless because neither he nor Ann Washkansky knew what the other meant by "chance." Did it mean Louis' chances of surviving the operation itself, or surviving a few weeks, months, or years

after the operation, or of better prospects with or without the operation? Furthermore, "an 80 percent chance" was indefensibly optimistic for any of these categories, given the fact that the operation
had never before been performed. Barnard's answer only served the
purpose of stopping any self-reflection by doctor or patient and of
deflecting any disturbing inquiries by and conversation with Ann
Washkansky.

To return to Blaiberg's story, here is Barnard's account of their
first meeting:

> I . . . went down to D-I Ward where I found Dr. Blaiberg dozing
> in bed. He looked like Santa Claus, with a tubby belly, red
> cheeks, blue ears, and a big mouth—except this was no laugh-
> ing Santa. His mouth was open and gasping for air.
>
> I nudged him slightly, and he looked at me with elfish eyes.
> "Dr. Blaiberg? I've come to introduce myself—or do you
> know who I am?"
> "No, I don't."
> "I'm Professor Barnard."
> "I'm sorry, Professor . . ."
> He gasped for air and continued.
> "I should have recognized you . . . I've seen your pictures
> often . . . but we've never met."
> "Well, I've come to say hello and see how you are."
> "You can see . . . I'm not well."
> In a way, he was worse off than Washkansky had been—
> especially, in the struggle for air.
> "Do you know there's a possibility we can help you by doing
> a heart transplant on you?"
> "Yes, I know."
> "How do you feel about that?"
> "The sooner, the better . . . I'll co-op . . . cooperate in
> every way."
> I looked into his eyes to see if there was fear. There was
> none. This was not a fighter like Louis Washkansky. He was
> not a loner. He was a company man—one of many. But he was
> without fear, and he believed that we could do it.
> "Good," I said. "I'll come again soon."
> "Thank you, Professor . . ."
> He began to cough and I waited for him to finish.
> "The sooner . . . the better," he said.
> I returned to my office in the medical school. . . .

Having established by a look into Blaiberg's eyes that there was no fear and by another unidentified process that he was a "company man"—by which Barnard must have meant that Blaiberg had "the interests of the employer rather than those of the workers at heart"[4] and therefore would loyally follow orders—Barnard seemed satisfied. Neither Barnard's nor Blaiberg's reminiscences mention any further conversations between them about the impending heart transplantation.

Barnard's initial conversation with Louis Washkansky, although somewhat more extensive than the one with Blaiberg, was equally devoid of any exploration of their respective expectations, fears, and hopes. Dr. Kaplan, Washkansky's family physician, had urged Barnard to explain the heart transplant operation to Washkansky and this was one of the ostensible reasons for his first visit. According to Barnard, he found Washkansky "propped up in bed, reading a book":

> "Mr. Washkansky, I have come to introduce myself. I believe Dr. Kaplan and Professor Schrire have spoken to you about it— we intend doing a heart transplant on you, and for this you will be admitted to my ward."
>
> "That's fine with me—I'm ready and waiting for it."
>
> "If you like, I can tell you what we know and what we don't know about this."
>
> He nodded and waited for me to go on. He was obviously very sick, but you could see he had once been quite strong and good-looking. There were also the features of a generous man—a large mouth with the face folds of one who smiled often. He had big ears and big hands, and his eyes, peering at me over the spectacles, were gray-green—and waiting. So, I spoke to him.
>
> "We know you have a heart disease for which we can do nothing more. You have had all possible treatment, and you are getting no better. We can put a normal heart into you, after taking out your heart that's no longer any good, and there's a chance you can get back to normal life again."
>
> "So they told me. So I'm ready to go ahead."
>
> He said no more. His eyes remained on me but with no indication he wanted to know any more.
>
> "Well, then . . . good-bye," I said.
>
> "Good-bye."
>
> As I turned to go, he began reading again. It was a Western. How, I wondered, could he return to pulp fiction after being suddenly cast into the greatest drama of his life? What was it about human nature that caused such a reaction? No man in

the history of the world had ever met the surgeon who was going to cut out his heart and replace it with a new human one—at least, not until this moment, which was now being lost somewhere in a Western novel.

What had made him turn away? He was a realist. He carried no false illusions, no special clouds of rationale. He lived for the moment, for the hour, for the full living of all of it. And now, I had offered him just that—life. Yet he had not asked the odds, nor any details.[5]

Washkansky's apparent disinterest in learning more about the operation disturbed Barnard momentarily. However, he brushed aside his concerns over Washkansky's puzzling behavior and concluded instead that "nothing more, no words were needed."

Should Barnard have insisted that more was needed, that they had to talk with one another so that both would know, for example, that he was offering Washkansky only the possibility, but surely no promise, of life? Should he have insisted that they talk more, particularly in this instance, since "no man in the history of the world had ever met the surgeon who was going to cut out his heart"? Should he have inquired why Washkansky who would soon come face to face with the "greatest drama of his life" returned "to pulp fiction"?

In raising these issues, I do not question that ultimately Washkansky might have made the same choice. I only question the nature and quality of Barnard's and Washkansky's thinking about available choices. Both, at best, had reflected on the forthcoming operation in isolation, and neither had any idea what had transpired in the other's mind. At the least, respect for Washkansky's psychological autonomy required Barnard to challenge his patient's silent acquiescence. In this case, where the patient was especially needy and was surrounded by seemingly powerful healers, his hopes, fears and magical expectations should not have been left unexplored.

If Washkansky wanted a new heart, he also had to have the heart to learn more about the operation. The first heart transplant was an extraordinary procedure. In selecting an appropriate patient, Barnard needed to pay attention not only to Washkansky's physical suitability for undergoing the operation but also to Washkansky's capacity to understand the consequences. Any patient who did not meet the latter criterion was not a suitable candidate for the first transplanted heart. In more ordinary situations . . . a patient's waiver of disclosure and consent may be more acceptable after a prior inquiry into his reasons. Washkansky's operation, however, was not an ordinary event. The inattentiveness to conversation in this instance, which made meaningful consent impossible, only underscores its general disregard in physician-patient interactions.

The silence about airing important concerns on the part of both parties is strikingly illustrated in Barnard's second meeting with Blaiberg. Washkansky had died in the meantime and Barnard asked for Blaiberg's help in "taking up another plane . . . to get back my confidence." Barnard apparently did not ask himself first whether his patently self-interested request—particularly the way he expressed it—was an appropriate one. Should he have known that unless he carefully distinguished between his interests and those of his patient, neither he nor Blaiberg could ever be sure whether consent to the surgery was given more for Blaiberg's own sake or for that of Barnard and his team? One example of such confusion is Blaiberg's statement that he wanted to go through with the operation because Barnard had already put so much "effort [into saving] Louis Washkansky."

While the rational and irrational expectations and their impact on the interactions between Barnard, Washkansky and Blaiberg clearly emerge in their personal reminiscences of their meetings, these expectations were never identified; they were passed over in silence. The process of thinking about choices was given all too short shrift. Thus another question arises: To what extent must physicians as well as patients subject their motivations and expectations to reflection and critical appraisal prior to and during their encounters?

Barnard's reminiscences give no indication that he engaged in self-reflection in order to sort out his conflicts of interest. He did admit to being severely shaken by Washkansky's death and to guilt. He told both Blaiberg and his friend and fellow-surgeon Jacques Roux, "I crash-landed." Indeed, Barnard entertained the idea of not performing another heart transplant. He did not consider sharing his doubts with Blaiberg, however, when he finally decided to proceed and went to Blaiberg to ask for his help.

Immediately after Washkansky's death, Barnard briefly withdrew into himself. Roux's comforting words that he "had opened the way for others" did not console him. Instead, he accused himself:

> No, Jacques, we crashed because of my mistakes. I should not
> have used cobalt treatment. I gave too many antirejection
> drugs. He got an infection because we lowered his resistance
> too much. And we didn't correctly diagnose that, until too
> late. . . . Even with what we know now, it'll still be working in

the dark and I've lost my nerve. I'm afraid, Jacques. I'm afraid of the dark.

At the subsequent autopsy, still depressed over his failure, Barnard's spirits lifted quickly once the pathologist pointed to the implanted heart:

"Chris," he said. "These suture lines are perfect—there's not an error or a clot anywhere. It's beautiful."

I looked from him to the other faces around the table. Each one nodded, or in some way said to me: "Well done, Chris."

At that moment I had my answer and I began to build again. I had not failed. I had succeeded. The first attempt, with all its pain and sorrow, had been made for the second. To now turn back would be to deny the first—*to turn away from Louis Washkansky's dream.*

Leaving the postmortem with Jacques, I said I was going to do another transplant.

"What's more," I said, "I'm going to America and appear on 'Face the Nation.' I'm going to face the world—and then come back and do a transplant on Dr. Blaiberg."

"Provided Dr. Blaiberg is still willing," said Jacques.

"Yes," I said. "And I'd better *find that out* right now."

When I reached the ward Dr. Blaiberg was awake, and his wife, Eileen, was sitting with him. . . .

*   *   *   *

"Dr. Blaiberg, do you know that Mr. Washkansky died this morning?"

"No, I didn't know it."

"I didn't tell him," said his wife. "I didn't know how to tell him."

"I expected it," he said. "I've been listening to the radio . . . I knew how ill he was."

"I've come to tell you why he died and what we found on examining him."

Dr. Blaiberg nodded and his wife held his hand.

"He died of pneumonia, and there was no evidence, as far as we could see, of a failure of the transplanted heart. But the transplant was a failure anyway, because we kept him alive for only eighteen days. So if you don't want to have your operation, you don't have to go through with it. It's for you to decide."

"Professor . . ."

He stopped to glance at his wife, then continued.

"I want to be a well man, and if I'm not well, I'd rather be dead. How soon can you do the next transplant?"

"Thank you."

"How soon can you do it?"

"I have to go overseas for about ten days, but we'll do it as soon as possible after I come back. In the meantime, I'll have you transferred to my ward."

"More than ever," he said, "I want this to be a success—not only for my sake, but also for you and the other doctors."

"You can help us by doing one thing."

"Yes—what is it?"

"Stay alive until I get back."

"Don't worry," he said. "You'll find me here—waiting."

Barnard's depiction of his goal as fulfilling "Washkansky's dream" is startling and suggests that he was as confused about his identity as Blaiberg was about his own. The dream that now propelled Barnard to go on was no longer his, but Washkansky's! Barnard's difficulty in distinguishing himself from Washkansky probably was influenced by guilt and sadness over Washkansky's death and by a wish to bring him back to life intrapsychically by making a common cause with "Washkansky's dream." At the same time he also must have been angry at Washkansky for having abandoned him—a common grief reaction among mourners who have lost an important person. He displaced his anger onto Blaiberg by abandoning him for ten days in order to "Face the Nation." Even though Barnard's trip to New York was motivated by other reasons as well, it may not be too far fetched to speculate that his anger at Washkansky for dying played a role in his leaving Blaiberg at this crucial moment.

Let me offer another speculation: Barnard may also have needed proof that Blaiberg would turn out to be a better patient than Washkansky, by "[staying] alive until [he got] back." If Blaiberg could accomplish that feat then perhaps he would stay around longer after the operation than Washkansky had. If this speculation has merit, it only proves that physicians are not exempt from magical thinking.

The needs and wishes of Barnard, Blaiberg and even a dead Washkansky became hopelessly intertwined in Barnard's mind. In Barnard's and his patients' dreams about the operation, an identity of interest could readily be taken for granted. If their dreams had been subjected to the harsh reality of waking thought, however, their conflicting interests would have become apparent. Guided too much by dreams, Barnard remained unaware of the potential conflicts between his own interests and those of his patients. Had he paused and reflected, he might have been able to separate his interests from theirs as they affected his thinking about the available choices as well as about the ultimate decision. Since he did not, he could neither explore them with himself nor consider informing Blaiberg about his doubts about the operation that he had shared earlier with his friend Roux.

Like so many physicians, Barnard assumed that his interests were the same as those of his patients and thus felt no hesitation to acting on behalf of Washkansky and Blaiberg. Respect for their psychological autonomy, however, would have demanded that Barnard keep his and their identities separate in order to explore their individual hopes and fears about the operation. Some might contend that the patients' necessitous and precarious conditions made any committed effort by Barnard to explain himself and his operation futile and irrelevant. The patients' self-inflicted coercions and magical expectations, however, must also be evaluated in terms of Barnard's contribution to the final outcome. His silence about crucial matters and his own magical expectations about the operation powerfully affected his patients' choices. Recall, for example, that Barnard told Blaiberg and his wife that Washkansky had "died of pneumonia, and [that] there was no evidence, as far as we could see, of a failure of the transplanted heart." Yet to his friend Roux he had spoken of "still working in the dark," of having given "too many antirejection drugs," and of having "lowered [Washkansky's] resistance too much."

Necessitous conditions notwithstanding, Barnard should at least have made an effort to inform his patients about what he knew and did not know about heart transplant operations and then to identify and clarify any misconceptions and distortions in their responses to his invitation of joining him in this great adventure. Even if his patients had initially resisted his invitation to converse and think together, Barnard should have insisted that they talk for a while. The inevitable conflict that such insistence creates between the values of autonomy and privacy should be resolved in favor of autonomy. Such invasions of privacy must be tolerated in order to enhance patients' psychological autonomy through insight and not allow it to be further undermined by too hopeful promises, blind misconceptions, and false certainties.

John Stuart Mill's words bear repeating: "Considerations to aid his judgment, exhortations to strengthen his will, may be offered to him, even obtruded on him, by others: but he himself is the final judge."[6] Mill appreciated the need for conversation. Respect for psychological autonomy finds expression in the first part of Mill's recommendation, in being attentive to the vulnerabilities of the process of thinking about choices. Respect for individual rights finds expression in Mill's second assertion that patients' ultimate choices must be honored. These distinctions . . . may clarify the common clinical controversy over whether physicians should respect either patients' "*rights*" or "*needs*." Insisting on conversation and reflection expresses a concern for patients' needs. The ultimate acceptance of their choices expresses a respect for their rights.

NOTES

All unidentified citations in the text refer to the last preceding source marked in the notes.

1. Blaiberg, P., *Looking at My Heart* (New York: Stein and Day, 1968), pp. 65–66.

2. Fox, R. and Swazey, J., *Courage to Fail* (Chicago: University of Chicago Press, 1974), p. 111.

3. Barnard, C. and Pepper, C., *Christiaan Barnard: One Life* (New York: Macmillan, 1969), pp. 260–61, 360, 392–93.

4. *Webster's New International Dictionary*, unabridged. 2nd ed. (Springfield, Mass.: G. & C. Merriam Company, 1959).

5. Barnard and Pepper, *supra* note 3.

6. Mill, J., *On Liberty* (London: John W. Parker & Son, 1859).

EDITOR'S NOTE

Dr. Katz, scheduled to present a paper and lead a discussion on informed consent, unfortunately became ill on the eve of the conference. This excerpt from his book, which fully explores the importance of physician-patient dialogue in preserving the autonomy and self-determination of the patient, represents a springboard from which conference discussions of the informed consent process between Barney Clark and his surgeons would have taken place, had Dr. Katz been able to attend. In allowing permission to reprint this excerpt, Dr. Katz intends no similarities between the informed consent process for the first two cardiac transplant patients, Louis Washkansky and Philip Blaiberg, and the consent given by Barney Clark.

Dr. Katz has given us a glimpse of what transpired between Dr. Christiaan Barnard and his first two heart transplant patients in December 1967 and January 1968. Since that time, much attention has been paid to the principles of disclosure, patient autonomy, self-determination, and informed consent. Court cases have delineated for the medical profession the contours of informed consent in the therapeutic setting, and the federal government has established guidelines for informed consent in human experimentation. It may be illuminating, then, to consider the informed consent process in Dr. Barney Clark's case, fifteen years after the South African experiences.

In the Utah heart implant case we have an extensive informed consent document available, approved by the University of Utah Institutional Review Board (IRB) and signed twice by Dr. Clark (see Appendix A). This form includes disclosures about the alternative procedure of heart transplantation (section 1.2), the possible need to repair or replace the artificial device (section 2.2), and the possible necessity of further invasive procedures (section 2.3); warns of unforeseen conditions during surgery (section 3), foreseeable and unforeseeable complications (section 5), the experimental nature of the procedure (section 6.1), and the limits of animal experimentation (section 6.2); expresses no guarantees (section 7) as well as an offer to answer questions (section 8, and repeated at the end of the document); and discusses life expectancy (section 10), cardiac assist pumps (section 12), and extended hospitalization (section 13). What we don't know is the subjective content of the conversations that preceded Dr. Clark's consent. We do, however, know something about the activities of the participants.

Barney Clark had been referred to Dr. Jeffrey Anderson, a cardiologist at the University of Utah Medical Center, by Dr. Terence Block, a cardiologist in Seattle, for treatment of idiopathic myocardopathy with progressive congestive heart failure, two and one-half years earlier. His condition was managed medically, including administration of digoxin, furosemide with potassium supplementation, warfarin, captopril, prednisone, azathioprine, and a trial of the investigational new inotropic drug amrinone, all of which proved unsuccessful in preventing further cardiac decompensation. The diagnosis was established by electron microscopic examination of a cardiac biopsy.

Six weeks prior to implantation, Dr. Anderson referred Barney Clark to the surgical implant team for evaluation of his candidacy for an artificial heart. After a visit to the animal barn, where he and Mrs. Clark were shown animals with heart implants and engaged in lengthy discussions with Dr. William DeVries, the surgeon, and Dr. Donald Olsen, the veterinary pathologist, concerning prognosis, risks, benefits, and alternative treatments, he was discharged from the hospital and given a copy of the approved IRB consent form to take with him on his return to Seattle. Thus, he was not in the potentially coercive atmosphere of the hospital when he made his decision. He discussed the pros and cons with his family, his friends, and his Seattle cardiologist, but he stated that the final decision was his alone to make. After considering his options in the face of further clinical deterioration, he requested readmission for implant surgery.

He returned to the hospital two days before the operation. The six members of the heart subcommittee of the IRB talked with him individually and gave final unanimous approval. After reading and lengthy discussions, Dr. Clark signed the consent form twice, with an interval of twenty-five hours between signatures. During that interval Dr. DeVries and Dr. Ross Woolley, a member of the IRB subcommittee, reviewed each paragraph in the consent document with him, offered to answer any further questions he might have, and attempted to determine that his consent was truly informed.

In his private diary, Dr. Woolley wrote the following description of the events that took place before Dr. Barney Clark signed the informed consent document the second time:

> Dr. DeVries and I met with Dr. Clark and went over the informed consent document again as required by the protocol. It was read word-for-word to him while he read along. There were a number of times when Dr. DeVries paused and asked him again if he understood the implications of the document. In all cases he responded in the affirmative. For example, when Dr. DeVries read paragraph 16 which states that the patient is free to withdraw his consent to participate, Dr. Clark responded by saying that if he did there would certainly be a lot of "long faces," followed by a smile and laugh. It is my firm judgment that to the greatest extent possible that Dr. Clark was fully cognizant of what he was signing and aware, to the extent that anyone could be, of the risks of the procedure. He signed the consent form for the second time at 9:52 P.M. on November 30, 1982.

The lengthy discussions between surgeon and patient, which Dr. Katz advocates, thus took place. It is not known, however, to what extent Dr. Clark was aware of Dr. DeVries' hopes and doubts about this first experiment. Dr. Clark stated many times after surgery, however, that he was glad to be able to contribute to medical research and hoped his experience would benefit future patients. He was certainly not under the misconception that the first experimental trial was being offered to him under the guise of therapy per se. To the extent possible, and under the circumstances of his impending death, I believe that Barney Clark's consent was autonomous, voluntary, and fully informed.

How Is the Death of Barney Clark to Be Understood?

ERIC J. CASSELL

INTRODUCTION

The impact of any death cannot be discussed in some global, overarching manner but must be viewed from a number of different perspectives. The failure to keep frameworks of reference separate in thinking about death and the care of the dying leads to much confusion. Consideration must be given to the dying body; the person who is dying; the two-person relationships, if any, of which the dying person is a part; the patient's family; the community; and sometimes, as in the case of Barney Clark, the nation and the world at large.

Each of the levels on which a death has an impact is distinctly separate from others, and each, despite obvious and necessary interrelationships, requires different information and kinds of understanding. The death of Barney Clark illuminates each of these levels. Despite the seeming abstractness of this approach to the care of the dying and the impact of a death, the death of Barney Clark makes clear the very practical consequences of disregarding them and of our ignorance of them.

Before going further, I believe it is necessary to make clear where I stand in regard to the artificial heart. There is no question that the amount of money being used to produce and implant the artificial heart could improve the health of many more individuals if it were employed for preventive services. But that, and many other objections that are raised against the advance of high technology are, to me, beside the point. Technology advances whether one agrees or not. One can turn aside or join, but as has been frequently noted, technology has its own imperative. Personally, I enjoy it. However, it seems reasonable that a new advance like the artificial heart, as discontinuous from previous capabilities as it is, should not be deployed in technological or scholarly isolation, so I sincerely applaud the openness of the Utah team and its willingness to explore so many issues connected to the device.

Unfortunately, when new technologies are developed, the focus of intellectual attention comes to be almost exclusively on the technology itself rather than on its impact on the surrounding world. For example, the artificial heart is implanted to avert a patient's death. But despite the attention death or its avoidance receives, whether the patient lives or dies may turn out to be only one of the fundamental issues raised by the implantation of the heart. Consideration of problems surrounding the care of the dying patient or of death itself, such as the levels I noted and on which I will be expanding, requires as much innovative thinking, research, and development as the heart implant itself. Perhaps the time has come to require an impact statement before radically new technologies such as this are further.implemented in order to prepare the society for the widespread effects of the new advance.

THE BODY

Although medicine concerns itself with the human body, its knowledge and its methodologies are most often directed at individual organs or subordinate levels of organization such as cells or even molecules. Except in the minds and actions of individual physicians responsible for patient care, rarely is this biological information integrated into knowledge about whole bodies. Put another way, bodily function or even single organ function is not frequently viewed as a whole. This deficiency of understanding has had little adverse effect in the development of artificial organs before the artificial heart, because despite the name, organs were not being replicated, biological functions were. For example, artificial blood is not blood at all; it is artificial oxygen-carrying capacity. Blood, as we all know, has many other functions besides oxygen transport. Similarly, the artificial hip is not a hip. It is not even a joint. It merely serves the function of articulation. Joints also have tendons, muscles, and capsules. Even the artificial kidney replaces only one function of the kidney—a permeable membrane in an exchange bath—while the natural kidney performs other tasks as well. Generally speaking, then, success has followed where a function has been replaced.

In listening to the manner in which people, including doctors, talk about artificial organs, one might come away with the belief that all the organs just sit there doing their own thing and that from that concert of individual actions, the function of the whole organism occurs. I was led to believe that the same viewpoint was, at least initially, held by the Utah team, because when Dr. Clark died, it was reported that his artificial heart had worked fine, but that his kidneys and his lungs did not hold up because they were so diseased prior to the implant. While I have no question that Barney Clark's kidneys and lungs were impaired after his long history of congestive heart failure, the failure of the body after the implant can be attributed to a failure of the implanted heart. It might have been a great heart while it was sitting in a box or on a test bench in splendid isolation, but it was not a good "Barney Clark Heart." To be a good "Barney Clark Heart," a heart had to have a very low cardiac output. Since we usually consider a good heart to be one with a high output, how is it that a good "Barney Clark Heart" should have a low output? Because all the organs of his body had adapted to the low output of his chronically failing heart. So had Barney Clark himself, and that adaptation takes time to change. If a new heart with the capacity for a high output is implanted, the "normal" output will have to be achieved slowly enough to give the other organs time to adapt and probably after starting at the output of the heart that has been replaced. We all know about how slowly the body adapts to the return of function of a previously diseased part. That adaptation is convalescence from the deconditioning that accompanies illness. But deconditioning is not deterioration except from an organ point of view. From the whole body framework of reference, it is adaptation to an enforced state of illness. After all, it would not do to have peak muscle strength coupled with a mind bursting with eagerness in a body that has a heart that cannot exceed two liters of output.

The problem of fitting the output of the artificial heart to the system in which it is being implanted will, predictably, be present every time the device is employed. Therefore, in the course of the care of the next patients who receive artificial hearts, information can be obtained that will lead to an understanding of how whole bodies adapt to the change of a part. Such research will be important in itself, but it might also serve as a badly needed model for research on whole organisms. General systems theory has provided a manner in which to view problems of this sort, but a methodology robust enough for good systems research in humans is lacking.

Another practical consequence of not realizing that the function of the artificial organ must be fitted to the system into which it is implanted has to do with what the patient and the family are told about the reasons for difficulties. As noted above, it was said that Barney Clark's new heart did not do as well as it might because of preexisting pulmonary disease. His chronic obstructive pulmonary disease was attributed, correctly, I am sure, to his prior cigarette smoking. But the implication is that the failure was really the fault of Barney Clark and his bad habits. It is my opinion that patients are all too ready to take the blame for failures, blame that their families come to share. The feeling of culpability remains long after the death and long after the words have left everybody else's mind. Attribution of blame is best left unsaid.

THE PERSON

Barney Clark died, not his body. Further, a sick Dr. Barney Clark died, not only Dr. Barney Clark who happened to have a diseased body. Although both statements may seem to be truisms, they contain distinctions that are often forgotten. Virtually everyone who has ever witnessed death or cared for the dying has tried to solve the puzzle of what disappears in the change of state from alive to dead. The attempt to make of the transition a simple biological matter has led to some strange writings. For example, Marie-François-Xavier Bichat in *Recherches Physiologiques sur la Vie et la Mort*, published in 1800, examined the changes that occurred postmortem in order to understand better what happens at death and the order in which the organs die. The book is an example of the sterility of the enterprise. Nonetheless, in applying the recent advances of medicine, it often appears as though it is merely the body that doctors must save from death.

In fact, of course, life makes a difference to persons. I presume that Dr. Clark underwent the discomforts and dangers of having the implant because he wanted to live rather than because he wanted to avoid dying. The distinction is important because it is often difficult for physicians, particularly young ones, to realize that there are things worse than death. When Jehovah's Witnesses refuse transfusions, even though death may be inevitable without the blood, they are not choosing to die. They are avoiding the far worse fate of having their souls condemned to everlasting purgatory because of the sin of receiving blood. When the patriot says "Give me liberty or give me death," he is implying that life without liberty is not worth living. Similarly, when a person with chronic kidney disease decides to discontinue renal dialysis despite the fact that death will follow, that person makes the choice that an existence of continued dialysis is intolerable, not that death is good. It is crucial to understand this for many reasons, but one of them is the confusion over the moral difference between starting and stopping a life-prolonging intervention. We are all aware that Dr. Barney Clark had to give permission for the implantation of the heart. If he had wished it discontinued after a time, he would not be committing suicide, he would be withdrawing permission for the intervention, presumably because life as "Barney Clark–plus–artificial heart" might have become more problematic than death as Barney Clark.

The foregoing is the reason that many who regularly care for the dying believe that death may be important, but it does not matter as much as other things—living, for example. Such statements often sound strange to the healthy. After all, being not-living seems to be the same as being dead. Aside from the biological obviousness that if you are alive you are not dead, living is not at all the same as merely not dying. The focus of attention for the living (as "living" is meant here), especially those for whom the threat of death is immediate, is on the present and the important things contained in the present. Most healthy people spend very little time in the present, dwelling instead on future hopes, anticipations, fears, and distresses, and are guided more by their past than their present needs. It is difficult to get healthy individuals to focus on life in the present, which often sounds like some kind of hocus-pocus. But the very sick understand, or can be helped to understand, very much more easily. Thus far, at least, only sick people are candidates for artificial hearts, and so these concepts apply to them. So it is essential that in caring for those who receive heart implants, the staff places its emphasis on living, not on the avoidance of dying.

What I have just said may be denied by the fears for their continued existence that the very sick often exhibit. Indeed, their tendency to have many fears is striking. However, it is in the management of those fears by doctors and other caregivers that the very sick are freed to savor life in ways that make the sickness endurable or even better. But to deal with the fearfulness of the ill, one must realize that the sick are different from the well. They are not merely well people with a sickness appended to their sides, but in their relations to themselves, objects, and people, as well as their mechanisms of thought, they differ from the healthy. Knowledge of the characteristics of sickness, no matter which disease has imposed the state, is important to the care of heart implant recipients whether they live or die. Such characteristics cannot be considered the psychological aspects of the case, to be dealt with by psychiatrists or social workers, but must be understood as central to understanding how to deal with the diseased body as well.

In discussions such as this, reference is often made to the problems raised by the mind-body dualism. It is true that Cartesian dualism has outlived any utility it may have had, but here I am speaking of the body-person distinction. We all think of ourselves as persons, but the category of person has trouble finding a home (except in the law). Clearly a body is not a person, because person includes body. Mind is not a person, either. Person is a larger category than mind. Further, the notion of person—what it is to be a person—is different in different cultures and at different times. See how individualized— me, myself, and I—the idea of person is now compared with, say, what it was at the turn of the century. The distinction between body and person is clarified and its importance underlined by the problem of suffering.

Medicine's goal is often believed to be the relief of suffering. Indeed, the problem of human suffering is central to my theologies. But there is little understanding of what the word *suffering* means. If one searches the medical literature, one quickly notes that suffering and pain are usually linked, as in the expression "pain and suffering." But it is a simple matter to demonstrate that pain and suffering, although they are often found together, are discrete phenomena. For example, suffering may be caused by severe pain. I have recurrent renal colic, which, although it is very painful, is not a source of suffering to me. I know what is causing the pain, and I know that it can be relieved. Childbirth can be very painful, but modern methods of ameliorating the pain focus not on its absolute ablation but on giving the mother control over her own childbirth. On the other hand, patients may suffer greatly from rather mild pain if its source is unknown but suspected to be dire. Similarly, never-ending pain may cause suffering even though it is not severe. (Doctors and healthy people do not know much about this because people with endless pain learn not to say anything. What can you say after you have said it hurts?) The evidence that it is not the pain itself that causes the suffering is that suffering may be relieved in the foregoing situations by naming the pain and showing its source to be benign or by showing the patient that the pain can be controlled. In this second instance, after patients are aware that their pain can be relieved, they are often quite willing to tolerate it rather than to suffer from the side effects of the drugs. The distinction between pain or other physical symptoms and suffering is highlighted by the fact that one can suffer without any physical symptoms. Watching one's child in pain is a familiar example. I could adduce more evidence to show that suffering can arise from the loss of intactness or the threat of the dissolution of person in any of its many dimensions and that suffering can be relieved if the threat is ameliorated or intactness restored. But the basic point that is relevant here is that bodies do not suffer, persons suffer. If this is the case, then it is necessary to understand the nature of "person" in all its dimensions. These include the personality and character; the past that has been lived; the family's past; the impact of culture and society; relationships with others; roles; relationships with the body; the unconscious mind; day-to-day behaviors; the political existence; a belief in the future; a secret life; and last but by no means least, the transcendant dimension of being a person. It is in relationship to these aspects of being a person that suffering occurs (and may be caused by medical intervention as well as disease), and it is only in relation to them that suffering may be helped. Death is not important to bodies, only to persons.

We have seen, thus far, that the scientific view of artificial heart implantation deals primarily with units of the body—organs and their constituents—not with whole bodies or with the persons of whom the body is a part. This framework of reference can compromise the success of an implant unless the function of the artificial heart is fitted to the whole system of which it becomes a part. Further, the success of a procedure has to do primarily with the sick person who receives the implant, not merely that person's body. We have also seen how little is known, in a systematic manner, about persons. But it is important to realize that this lack of systematic knowledge of persons is not something that can be remedied by further scientific exploration of the subject (now that we realize how important it is). In fact, no modification of the current scientific viewpoint will or can encompass those aspects of persons that we might all agree are important (perhaps using ourselves or the Golden Rule as a guide). Witness the emptiness of most discussions of quality of life when they occur as part of clinical or scientific papers. No method of science can produce systematic understanding of persons, because no scientific methodology can be expected to discover what modern science does not consider to exist in the first place—notions of quality (virtue or excellence) and value. Without such consideration of quality and value any concept of person is empty of meaning. Other aspects that are entailed by personhood, such as ambiguity, uncertainty, nondistinction, or even complex change over time, are also opaque to science.

ETHICS

The increasing consideration that the sick person (rather than merely the disease) has received in medicine has been paralleled by the growth of the discipline of bioethics. In fact, one of the basic roles of ethics in medicine has been to provide a formal structure through which respect for persons is expressed in research on human subjects, in the care of the dying, as well as in the everyday diagnosis and treatment of the sick. Respect for persons has found its most concrete outward expression in the understanding that nothing can be done to any patient without his or her consent. In terms of the care of the dying, respect for persons leads us to the awareness that the dying person has the almost absolute right to be allowed to refuse treatment and even to choose his or her mode of death within the constraints of fate and the law.

Notions of respect for persons, however, are somewhat vague. Who, after all, would profess disrespect for persons? Thus, *respect* is rarely the key term used in discussions of ethics in medicine. Instead, reference is made to the importance of autonomy. But being autonomous, having the ability to exercise freedom of choice, is only one aspect of being a person. Basing ethics so heavily in autonomy suffers from the same fundamental defect as implanting an artificial heart based almost solely on knowledge of hearts (rather than whole bodies). I believe I can illustrate this defect by reference to the consent form signed by Dr. Barney Clark prior to the artificial heart implantation. Consent forms, as they are increasingly being employed in medicine, are meant to provide the information about the risks, benefits, and alternatives to the procedure or treatment in question that would allow a prudent person to decide in his or her own best behalf. In order to meet this standard, the University of Utah Institutional Review Board (IRB) apparently considered it necessary to require a consent form that was eleven pages long. Further, Dr. Clark was to sign the consent on the occasion of his reading it (in company with his doctors who were to provide him with any further information that he might desire) and again twenty-four hours later. Finally, according to criteria established by the IRB, to be a suitable candidate for artificial heart implantation, a patient had to be near death from chronic congestive heart failure. It requires little clinical experience to know that sick persons cannot read and correctly comprehend eleven pages of technical information about the device that offers them their only hope of returning to life.

It seems reasonable to ask whether a hypothetical Dr. Barney Clark would have signed such a form, in an unknown place, peopled by faceless strangers, had he been sent there for a previously unknown kind of medical procedure, as ill as we know him to have been. The reason it seems unlikely that Dr. Clark or anyone else would sign under such circumstances is that the whole consent procedure is based on trust. Where trust is absent, consent, informed or otherwise, becomes extremely problematic. One knows this to be true because the information provided by consent forms is meant to reduce uncertainty and permit people to act in their own best behalf. The more crucial the action and the more dangerous the alternatives, the more intolerable uncertainty becomes and the more information that is required. But information can only be expected to reduce uncertainty if it is believable. To be believable, information must come from a trusted source. In life-and-death medical decisions, uncertainty can only rarely be reduced to zero. There is never enough information, if only because the future is involved. In such circumstances, individuals resort to trust in others to solve the problem presented by ineradicable uncertainty. Expert others not only have more information and knowledge, both latent and manifest, but they are considered to have the ability to make decisions involving competing probabilities. Deciding who to trust is a personal matter, but it is also social. Trust depends on the mutual obligations and responsibilities each of us has in relation to others because of our roles and relationships within the shared matrix of culture and society. Thus, the consent form given Dr. Clark to sign, and which stands as a tribute to the importance we place on autonomy, underlines the inadequacy of the concept of autonomy.

In the simplest terms, there is no autonomous, free-standing individual of the type pictured by currently dominant ethical theory. In the same manner, there is no isolated piece of matter, from mitochondria to muscle to hearts, as pictured by science. However, ideas about autonomous individuals and isolated matter have been extremely productive artificial constructions. Neither, unfortunately, is adequate to the artificial heart program. I am aware that despite the inadequacies of these concepts, there will be further progress because practical people generally discover practical solutions to practical problems long before they discover theoretical solutions. On the other hand, theory must ultimately change, or in its pursuit of progress society risks being trapped, instead, in repetitive, boring newness. An example of what I mean is provided by those forecasts about the future of medicine that detail the new technology just beyond the horizon. New technology is new in the sense that a 1984 model automobile is new, not in the more important sense of a new understanding of transportation that portends methods of transport that are currently unimaginable. The advances in theory that are required will show how autonomy is modified by the fact of other people, families, communities, and society, in general. For medicine, it is necessary to understand how a relationship with a doctor might promote, rather than limit, the patient's autonomy.

The next levels to be discussed, two-person dyads and the family, make even clearer the inadequacy of current concepts of autonomy as they apply to medicine.

RELATIONS BETWEEN TWO PERSONS

In exploring the consent procedure in this case, one might get the idea that the IRB believes that not only is Dr. Clark the only person who can decide what is in his best behalf but that in some way he must be protected from interference in that choice by his doctors or the medical center. There are commentators on bioethics who would state, putting the case more strongly, that Dr. Clark and his doctors are adversaries. Because it is generally conceded that beneficent motives are fundamental to the medical enterprise, in the usual instance, any actions that might be interpreted by some as interference in Dr. Clark's choices would be defended by his doctors as being in Dr. Clark's interest. In the bioethics literature, the derogatory term *paternalistic* is applied to physicians who think that they might know the interests of the patients better than the patients themselves do.

Somehow the charge of paternalism seems overly simple. Everyday experience suggests that on occasion, less swayed by physical symptoms, false expectations, inordinate desire, or unrealistic fears (to name but a few of the influences that may cloud the judgment of the sick), others may know our own best interests better than we. It is also well known that physicians can and frequently do act in the service of their patients without putting themselves or their own selfish interests above their patients. The nature of the bonds between pairs of people that promote selfless concern for one another are not well understood today. In previous times words like *selfless, trustworthy, honorable, altruistic, compassionate,* and similar morally descriptive terms were taken to represent real traits by which the sick or the weak might be protected or cared for by others. These moral bonds have become the subject for distrust, and in their place there has been erected a structure of law and regulation designed to accomplish the same goals with less bias and greater protection from human foibles. Despite their advantages, these technical substitutes for previous moral bonds are formed around median standards of behavior that do not, I believe, promote higher standards. Cramped by a world view that sees people as almost exclusively atomistic individuals, we remain surprisingly ignorant of the bonds that can form between two people and that cause them to behave well toward each other. Since the relationship between doctor and patient is such a bond, medicine is the poorer for the lack of understanding of physician-patient bonding. No regulation or consent procedures will protect the recipient of an artificial heart better than the obligations and responsibilities of those charged with his or her care. It is reasonable to explore what in the environment of medical care (in this instance, in the University of Utah Medical Center) promotes these bonds of responsibility and what hinders them. In pursuing this subject it is interesting to note how little is known in any systematic manner. In fact, one will learn more from literature, particularly the romantic poets, than from the fields of psychology or the social sciences.

THE FAMILY

Husbands and wives are the two-person relationships that first come to mind in the preceding context. But husbands and wives are not true dyads; they are members of a family. And a family, no matter how small, always presumes other people without whom there would be no family, at the very least those in the previous generation. Thus, the family is always in debt to the past. In addition, the family is always in thrall to the future because that is the expectation of families.

We are in the habit of considering the loss of a physical presence to be the phenomenon of greatest importance in any death, and in terms of the decedent that certainly must be true. But there are other changes that are as decisive and irretrievable. The death of an individual almost always changes the structure of a family. When Dr. Barney Clark died, his generation of his family died with him, his wife became a widow, and his children lost their father. The social (and personal) status of each of them changed, and that change is reflected in the way the world behaves toward them and the manner in which they behave toward themselves and toward each other.

The kind of medical care a person received prior to and at the time of death influences the changes that take place in the family. It was common in 1961 when I started practicing, in order to reduce the pain of the loss of a loved one, to shield the relatives from as much of the unpleasantness of death as possible. The standard practice at the time leads one to deduce that the received wisdom was that death is a permanent separation that should take place as cleanly and completely as possible and that once the physical cleavage has occurred, the worst is over. Or, to put it more bluntly, dead is dead;

let the living get on with life. Family members were often discouraged from long stays at the bedside during the patient's last days, although it was not rare for spouses, parents, or children to insist that they belonged there. The family was even more vigorously shielded from agonal sights and sounds. Young children were kept away from sickbeds, in general, and even more so from the dying. When families asked whether the children of someone about to die should be brought home from, say, college, it was often thought wise that the soon-to-be-bereaved should stay away and attempt to lead as normal a life as possible. The aged were protected from the knowledge of the impending death of a loved one for fear of the risk to their well-being posed by the bad news. The words *dead, dying,* or *death* were rarely used directly. Instead, euphemisms were employed. This further increased the distance between dying persons and their loved ones. These behaviors became popular at the same time that the scene of death shifted from homes to institutions. It should be noted, however, that twenty years ago, intensive care areas and very intrusive life-sustaining or resuscitation equipment was absent or rare.

Current beliefs about these issues highlight how much things have changed. Present understandings focus on the importance of behaviors occurring at the time of the separation of the living from the dead. It is as though the closure of relations between loved ones can occur in special ways at the time of death that are not possible (at least in the same manner) at other times in the life cycle. Further, more and more people believe that when such emotional resolution does not occur at the time of death, the lack can never be remedied, and the pain of grieving will be greater. Statements such as "I had a chance to tell my father I loved him, and this was very important to me" are typical of this belief.

As a consequence of these recent changes in attitudes, it is increasingly accepted that the care received by the dying patient should facilitate the resolution of relations between the patient and loved ones. For this to occur, several goals must be pursued. The first is to allow a smooth and emotionally complete separation at the time of death. The primary step toward this is facilitating communication between patient and loved ones so that both patient and family know, as much as possible, what is the diagnosis and when death is to be anticipated. In the case of Dr. Barney Clark, there was no lack of such information.

The physical setting also influences the opportunities for loved ones to be close to the dying patient. Consequently, increased length and convenience of visiting hours, open access of family to the patient's bedside, reduced intrusiveness of medical procedures and hospital bureaucratic concerns can all increase the ability of the family to visit the patient. Although many of these are not directly controlled by the physicians, they have considerable influence in individual instances. The vital fact that must be remembered is that the well-being of loved ones is part of the doctor's responsibility in terminal illness. Naturally, there are limits to that responsibility, and problems arise when the needs of the family and those of the patient conflict. I believe that, in such cases, the primary responsibility of physicians is to their patients. Here, as in other circumstances, compromise and open discussion often allow conflicts to be resolved. Doctors can help family members say good-bye in a smooth and fulfilling way when they understand the present belief that the family must be permitted to spend as much time as possible at a bedside, that saying good-bye is important for each loved one, and that whenever possible, it is best that spouse, parents, or children who wish should be allowed to be present at the time of death.

Unfortunately, many physicians view the needs of the family as obstacles to the essential activity of caring for the patient's illness. Although family needs may, on occasion, intrude, in the case of the dying patient the physician must set new goals that include the well-being of the surviving family. When the outcome is uncertain, as in experimental procedures such as artificial heart implantation, conflicting responsibilities may be more difficult to resolve. When a realistic chance at meaningful survival exists, current attitudes give the patient's body highest ultimate priority. In the instance of Dr. Clark and in future artificial heart implantations, the community and the nation also have needs that are met largely through the media. When the needs of the family and the world at large are in conflict, it seems clear that the family comes first. Inasmuch as the media frequently behave as though they are unaware of this principle, it must be reinforced by the physicians in charge.

In addition to facilitating a smooth separation from the dying patient, physicians should, as much as possible, help relieve survivors of the inevitable guilt that accompanies bereavement. Although the source of the guilt is unclear, its presence seems universal. Free-floating guilt seeks any event on which to fasten. Physicians have the opportunity to lessen the reality basis of survivors' guilt. The newly bereaved should leave the deathbed with the faith that they and the doctors have done the right thing for their loved ones. They should believe that nothing better could have been done, no better decisions made, no more consultations considered, and that even God would approve of the actions taken. Physicians should help diminish opportunities for survivors to blame themselves or the medical attendants. As was done in the care of Barney Clark, family members must be kept informed as the case progresses and be permitted to take part in decision-making whenever possible. Loved ones should understand the reasons for important medical actions and realize that physicians care as much about the relief of suffering as they do. The family should not be overprotected with undue optimism or false hopes. Rather, to the degree possible, they should be made aware of forthcoming risks and complications. Family rivalries often surface and intensify at the bedside of a dying parent. It is impossible for the doctor to solve the problems at a deathbed that have occupied the family for a generation. It is feasible, however, to insist that everyone be notified, that every family member have a chance to visit and say good-bye, and that everyone of the same family rank participate in or have access to the decision-making process, when possible. Great, and frequently thankless, diplomacy may be required in such situations, but it is better attempted than not.

While facilitating separation and removing as many reasons for future guilt as possible, the physician must take care not to overburden family members. Loved ones may see their own needs as selfish, or worse, compared with obligations to a dying person, which may be perceived as boundless. Limits should be placed on what is expected of family members and on the degree to which they will be exposed to painful sights, smells, and sounds. Because individuals vary in their ability to tolerate the physical unpleasantness of dying, there can be no hard-and-fast rules. One errs best on the side of protection, but then one should be as flexible as possible about the behavior of individual family members. The custom, followed in many hospice units, of giving the visitors one day off a week is a wise one and might guide physicians in their advice to the family. The aim is to avoid a spouse (or other family member) getting so worn out in advance that no reserve is left to cope with the death itself.

Like everyone else, the bereaved must organize experience according to categories that are consonant with culturally accepted views of reality. There are a number of things that are commonly experienced by the recently bereaved that are not encompassed by our culture's world view. Thus, a bereaved spouse who feels an extremely strong sense of postdeath presence—exemplified by "I would hear a sound in the bedroom and know she was calling me, that she needed something. Then I would go in, and of course she wasn't there"—may consider it a mental aberration. The prolonged pain of loss experienced by the bereaved may be attributed by themselves and others to abnormal grieving. Similarly, the continued dependence of the mourner upon the dead person and his or her advice ("I think, What would he tell me to do?") is often considered abnormal. When the bereaved find themselves experiencing the death and its aftereffects differently than they had expected or than is the culturally expressed norm, they may become isolated from the group, find their sense of wholeness threatened, their understanding of events undermined, and their ability to control the grieving process inadequate. These features, which are common concomitants of physical sickness, may in themselves become a potent force in promoting illness in the bereaved person.

Physicians can be a powerful force in resolving some of the difficulties that arise when survivors' experiences cannot be explained by culturally acceptable categories of reality. Physicians have an important normalizing function. We commonly return patients to peace with their world by considering normal what the patient feared was abnormal. In the care of the bereaved, physicians can serve the same normalizing function by validating those experiences that the survivor fears are abnormal or even a sign of craziness. In addition, doctors who have had sufficient experience can provide the reassurance that for this culture (as for all others) there are acceptable realities outside of the shared categories of society.

In summary, physicians can reduce the stress of bereavement by the way they provide care to the dying person, facilitating emotional resolution and separation, reducing the opportunities for guilt-producing behavior, and easing the physical and emotional burdens that accompany terminal illness. In addition, doctors can reduce the potential for illness by the manner in which they deal with the bereaved's experiences for which the usual categories of cultural reality may be insufficient.

When a physician attends a person whose terminal illness has been long, complex, or unusually dramatic, the relationship with the family may become particularly intense. The doctor, seen in the hospital regularly or visiting or calling the home frequently, becomes a temporary family member. For the soon-to-be-bereaved, the physician may be seen as a particularly strong and emotionally giving individual at a time when the family members' emotions are in turmoil and they are more aware of their weaknesses than their strengths. Following the death, if the doctor merely walks out, another loss has been sustained. It is important that some arrangement be made for follow-up with family members after the death. There are difficulties here, because the bereaved do not consider themselves ill. But despite the fact that such follow-up may require walking an emotional tightrope, particularly when the doctor and the bereaved are of different gender and close in age, it is an important service. It is obvious that physicians are rarely trained to deal with such issues.

Despite all the attentions given to the bereaved soon after the death, abnormal grieving may not become manifest for many months or even years, and even then the tools for intervention are not clear. The one step that physicians or any caregiver can take that will be helpful is to make the bereaved know, without question, that should they have need, the physician is there and, further, that the nature of the need is a personal matter and differs from individual to individual. The bereaved should not feel it necessary to have to become sick in order to receive attention. Despite my obvious uncertainty about how intervention by physicians is best accomplished, it seems clear that the function will be facilitated if the doctor sets the stage at the time of the death for the follow-up.

Of all the foregoing, ethics is as ignorant as science. Ethics has, however, one precept to guide behavior in the absence of systematic understanding—respect for persons, for their wishes, fears, desires, and concerns. Respect for persons leads inevitably to respect for families, whose relationships, loves, and conflicts existed long before the sickness and will continue long after the death when everybody else has left or lost interest.

THE COMMUNITY AND THE NATION

The intense and persistent interest of the media testifies to the fact that the impact of the artificial heart implantation was not confined to Dr. Clark and his family. Only speculation is possible about why the procedure was so important to the outside world. However, we are aware that the myths of our communities and nation about science, progress, nature, medical care, doctors, surgeons, researchers, courage, death, loss, tragedy, and many other areas are built, supported, or changed by events such as the artificial heart implantation. The question must be asked whether the research team should consider itself responsible in any way or in any magnitude for these more distant effects of its efforts. If the answer is yes, then considerable effort and money must be expended in research for which most medical teams are, to say the least, poorly prepared. If the answer is no, then what are the limits of responsibility in the development of radically different technologies? I am not arguing for an unlimited extension of responsibility but merely the recognition that placing a mechanical heart in an individual sick body is the beginning, not the end, of the matter.

CONCLUSION

The implantation of the artificial heart into Dr. Barney Clark, his subsequent illness, and his death are monuments to biology, human creativity, the dedication to others that marks medicine at its best, and the magnificence of the human spirit. The marvelous complexity of the body, sick persons, and the world in which they live is not mirrored in the medical or ethical theory that guides the minds and hands of scientists and physicians. The case of Dr. Clark thrusts into prominence these failures of understanding: about how whole bodies integrate the functions of their parts; about what persons are and how they relate to disease in their bodies; about the relationship of persons to each other; about the impact of sickness on families; about the importance to communities of science and technology and their promise for the future. The artificial heart program gives promise that these areas of exploration will receive the attention they require, so that in the future, medicine will not only treat the sick but understand them.

NOTE

This paper was supported in part by the Commonwealth Fund and by a Sustained Development Award for Ethics and Values in Science and Technology (NSF OSS 80-18086) from the National Science Foundation and the National Endowment for the Humanities.

Summary of Discussion on Ethical Perspectives

DENISE GRADY

INTRODUCTION

This conference was held at a most sensitive time for the University of Utah's artificial heart program. Even though seven months had passed since the death of Dr. Barney Clark, the university's institutional review board (IRB) had yet to give the medical team permission to try the heart in a second patient. Team members were eager to get the project moving again, but Dr. Donald Olsen, the veterinarian in charge of animal studies of the device, described the researchers' position with the board as "precarious." The issues that the IRB was apparently sorting out included several discussed on the first morning of the conference: selection of patients, informed consent, and the nature of suffering.

Patient selection has been a difficult issue ever since surgeon William DeVries first sought the review board's approval for implanting the artificial heart, early in 1981. One thing he and the board agreed on from the beginning was that the recipient had to be so close to death that he had virtually nothing to lose by having his own heart cut out. In September 1981, the board gave DeVries permission to proceed but only with one type of candidate: a surgical patient who could not be weaned from the heart-lung machine and who had already signed release forms for the implant operation. Psychologically, this was difficult. It forced DeVries to confront people scheduled for heart surgery with the possibility that they might die on the table. The requirement seemed sure to undermine some patients' confidence in the surgical team, and DeVries initiated such discussions with only a few patients. In any case, all came off the pump. Seven months passed without a candidate.

In the spring of 1982, DeVries asked the IRB to expand the criteria to include patients with "chronic, inoperable, end-stage progressive congestive heart failure." That summer, the board agreed. Barney

Clark consulted DeVries in October and then, almost two months later, near death, returned to Salt Lake City for surgery.

Was he the right candidate? On one hand, he apparently had nothing to lose; he was dying of cardiomyopathy. On the other hand, he had severe lung disease and had been ill for some time. The few months he gained from the operation were marked by one setback after another. Perhaps a less ill patient would have recovered better, survived longer, and revealed more about the limits of the artificial heart.

The medical team and the IRB have reexamined the selection criteria with Clark's painful course in mind. DeVries has suggested expanding the criteria to include stronger patients, perhaps those with less advanced congestive heart failure or those who have suffered massive coronaries, have no hope of survival, and whose families consent to an implant. But by the time of this meeting in October, the board still had given no sign of which candidates, if any, it would allow. (In January of 1984 the board granted the medical team permission to proceed with a second patient—a less ill one, as DeVries had requested—and to test a lightweight, more portable drive system. In June, the FDA approved a second implant.)

SELECTING PATIENTS FOR THE ARTIFICIAL HEART

Dr. Albert Jonsen, the first speaker at the conference, addressed these issues of patient selection, although only indirectly. He raised this question: Is the dominant purpose of experimentation on human beings to benefit the person on whom it is performed, or to gather data that may help future patients? Jonsen maintained that the ethical justification for clinical research in its early stages is mainly utilitarian—aimed at gathering data to improve care for future patients—and not necessarily beneficial to the subjects themselves. Experimenters who think otherwise delude themselves and may even impede their own scientific progress by choosing subjects who, though most likely to benefit from the experiment—or at least not be harmed by it—are also unlikely to yield the data needed to advance the field. Given this utilitarian objective, the subjects must be volunteers in the fullest sense. They must know and accept the reality that they will not be the beneficiaries.

The first discussant challenged this position. Quoting from a document, Alexander Capron asked Jonsen to react to a passage that began, "Although a cardinal principle of initial human trials should be that there be no implantation without the prospect of therapeutic benefit, ..." And yet, Capron noted, Jonsen had suggested that therapeutic considerations are a human weakness that researchers slip into or allow themselves to be deceived by.

Jonsen immediately recognized the document—and his own prose. He'd written the passage some ten years ago in a report from the National Heart, Lung and Blood Institute's assessment panel for the totally implantable artificial heart. "It shows I change," he said, and explained that a decade ago, he himself had been "somewhat deceived" into thinking research had to benefit each subject. But he changed his mind as a result of work on the National Commission for the Protection of Human Subjects, which struggled over the term "therapeutic research" and finally abandoned it, because research by definition is not therapeutic. Since then, Jonsen said, he has considered research "primarily a utilitarian enterprise." But it must be "guarded and hedged about by the principles of benefit and autonomy."

Depending on one's reaction to Jonsen's thesis, the comments of the Utah medical team either proved him wrong—or revealed that the team had fallen into the very trap he described. DeVries said that in Barney Clark's case, he had the "dubious distinction" of trying to decide these issues while he was taking care of Clark. As a researcher, he did want to get on with clinical trials, but for him as a physician "the most important thing really was the care of the patient. Our first concern was benefit, not utilitarianism." The first and most difficult thing DeVries had to face, he recalled, was Clark's reaction to his condition upon awakening: "How was he doing as a person? Had it been therapeutic? Had we not done harm? Not put something into his chest that caused terrible pain, prolonged agony, and death?" Another reason the Utah project couldn't be called utilitarian, DeVries said, was that the IRB had never allowed him "the luxury of putting the device into the patients in whom it would do the most good and test the device in the best way. The only patient we were allowed was one in whom the benefit clearly outweighed the risks—a patient who was almost dead."

Agreeing with DeVries, Dr. Stanley Reiser said that in medical research, "Once you cross the line to human beings, the first consideration should be benefit to the subjects." The second, he said, should be gaining new knowledge. Dr. Willem Kolff shared this view, Reiser said, recalling Kolff's statement before the conference that he wouldn't have dreamed of putting a machine into any patient unless that person could be happy or benefit in some way.

Although Jonsen agreed that the point is worth arguing, he emphasized that it is still not certain that the thing being tested—the artificial heart—is therapeutic. So at this point, he said, to call it therapeutic and talk about its benefits to the patient "may be exaggerated or hyperbole."

Much of what Jonsen said, according to University of Utah President Dr. Chase Peterson, reflected "a legitimate desire to avoid scientific paternalism. That is, people who are obliged and able to know more must be very cautious about the way they direct the lives of people who know less." Those who know more must also realize that "no one outside the mind of the patient can know what led that particular patient to his or her decision." He said Barney Clark apparently had two major considerations. They mirrored both the therapeutic and utilitarian principles Jonsen had described. First, Peterson said, Barney Clark had a scientific, experimentalist's mind and was intrigued by the opportunity to take part in an important experiment; second, Clark was pragmatic and "intrigued by the thought that he might get something out of it." Peterson argued that an intellectual dissection of the issues might overlook or even damage "the unitary notion that it's one patient making a decision based on unknown factors within that patient's mind." Still, Jonsen insisted, it's important that researchers analyze their goals and honestly acknowledge the problems they face in pursuing them.

The discussion shifted to another aspect of the criteria used to select recipients of the artificial heart. Capron read from Dr. Lawrence Altman's article in the 17 April 1983 *New York Times*, which quoted members of the surgical team as saying that the most important lesson they had learned from Barney Clark was that patients need a strong, supportive family. The article went on to describe another candidate, a forty-eight–year–old man who badly wanted an artificial heart but was turned down because no one in his family cared much "whether he lived or died." The assumption that a caring family is a requirement for success has never actually been tested, Capron said, and he therefore questioned the fairness of retaining it as a criterion unless it has been studied and proved valid.

This issue is being discussed as the government considers the funding of heart transplants and the establishment of selection criteria, Jonsen replied. The impression that patients benefit from strong family ties came initially from experience with kidney transplants, he said, adding that he didn't know if a randomized, controlled trial of the assumption had ever been carried out and that he couldn't imagine how one would go about conducting such a study.

Peg Miller, the social worker on the Utah team, said that her years of experience with dialysis patients had convinced her that those with good support systems fare better. Dr. Eric Cassell agreed and mentioned that an ongoing study at Columbia University involving two groups of patients—one with family, and one without—supports what he says everybody knows intuitively.

The Utah team's decision to make family support one of the selection criteria was indeed based on the experiences of dialysis patients and transplant recipients, according to DeVries. Moreover, he said, social criteria had become one of the most frequent grounds for disqualifying patients. The psychiatrist in the Utah group, Dr. Claudia Berenson, added that studies of patients with other long-term illnesses had provided considerable evidence of the need for family support. But later, after the meeting, she explained that in many cases the relatives themselves were not crucial but their relationships with the patient were, because they demonstrated the patient's ability to get close to other people and depend on them when necessary.

Nonetheless, Capron insisted that the supposition should be tested before it becomes a permanent part of the criteria for patient selection. Jonsen observed that scientific study of this issue would be a truly utilitarian experiment, because the researchers would have to select some subjects whom they expected to fare poorly.

The medical team may also rely on the patient's family for emotional support, said Dr. Renée Fox, and in that case the team's view of the family as necessary for success becomes a self-fulfilling prophecy. She urged members of the Utah group to ask themselves how much they had depended on the Clark family.

"I have never seen an adult bull visit one of our calves," said Dr. Robert Jarvik, referring to the University of Utah's animal studies on the artificial hearts he has designed, "and yet the calves do very well. They have no family support." Jarvik also referred to Kolff's experience, stating that the first patient to survive on dialysis was a Nazi sympathizer in a Dutch village who was hated by all her neighbors. Therefore, he agreed with Capron that the team should not let family support slip in as an untested criterion, because it is unfair to disqualify people simply because they have no families.

Dr. Gilbert Omenn also challenged the supposition about family ties. For one thing, he suggested, the Clark family was extraordinarily cooperative. Next time, the Utah team might not be so lucky. Omenn also doubted the validity of comparing artificial heart recipients to dialysis patients. "With renal dialysis," he said, "you have a very well-proven technology, and you expect the patient to go home and need support there." It's still not clear that any patient with the artificial heart will go home. So, he said, having the patient surrounded by concerned relatives "may not be best for determining if a technology works." Maybe someone without a family would be a better subject, he suggested, because there wouldn't be other people hovering around who might be problems, asking embarrassing questions, pestering the staff, losing faith in the program, or engaging in outside business ventures that capitalize on the patient's experiences.

Omenn urged the Utah researchers to "be a little more hard-nosed" in choosing patients. For example, had they considered implanting the device in brain-dead subjects for physiological studies? Jarvik replied that Dr. Jack Kolff (Willem Kolff's son) had, in fact, tried the device for as long as three days in a brain-dead subject in Pennsylvania, but that it was nearly impossible to sort out problems like diabetes insipidus and pulmonary edema, which nearly always crop up in such patients. "A valid experiment," Jarvik concluded, "but not necessary." DeVries added that this type of experiment has its own ethical problems, because it destroys a potential donor's heart and kidneys.

MEASURING THE EXPERIMENT'S SUCCESS

The next discussion period, following Cassell's talk, addressed not only questions he raised about suffering and informed consent but also some questions left over from the earlier session, as well as general comments and ethical questions about the artificial heart.

The first comment came from Joann Ellison Rodgers, who had interviewed eleven seriously ill heart patients at the time of Barney Clark's surgery. They said he was not a hero, just a man trying to live. All but one said they would do as Clark had done. The one who disagreed was a twenty-nine–year–old man who had undergone a heart transplant the year before. He said that if he had it to do over again, he would refuse the transplant because his quality of life was so poor.

As for evaluating the experiment on Barney Clark, Jonsen said his death should not be regarded as a failure. From the utilitarian viewpoint he described—and he quickly noted he was "not saying we should go from caring therapeutics to crass utilitarianism"—the only failure would have been to fail to get data for the next experiment. The researchers should not have expected Clark to live, Jonsen said: "They should have counted it as great good luck if he lived."

Peterson asked the nursing staff to comment, because he believed that while caring for Clark, *they* had also suffered greatly in the psychic sense Cassell described. Helen Kee, director of nursing, said the nurses had seen Clark as a "human being who was suffering and dying, though I don't think he had any pain. We didn't see him as just an experimental activity. Intellectually, we understood that it was a first experiment. But we still had those feelings that go with seeing someone die, and maybe we had a sense of failure, too."

"Did you feel that if it hadn't been for this experiment," Peterson asked, "he wouldn't have been suffering?"

Kee said no. Linda Gianelli, who is in charge of the coronary care unit at the Utah medical center, added that she and her colleagues were not shocked by Barney Clark's suffering; considering his condition, it was to be expected. "We see many coronary patients with complicated courses and long hospital stays," she said. The unique thing about Barney Clark was that he frequently asked the medical team if they were learning enough. This appeared to mean a great deal to him. After the discussion period, Clark's nurses said their experience with him had not soured them on the artificial heart; on the contrary, they were eager to get on with the next patient, and they were disappointed that the university's IRB had not given the team permission while everything they had learned was still fresh in their minds.

Altman questioned the appropriateness of even talking about Barney Clark's case in terms of failure or success: "When in the history of medicine has a first experiment of any kind ever been truly successful? I can't find any"—not heart transplants, dialysis, penicillin, or even insulin. He concluded that it is only fair to measure what is happening now against the historical record.

Nonetheless, Cassell wanted to know what criteria the Utah team had used to measure success in Clark's case. What if he had lived a year? DeVries replied that the entire team had discussed that question, and the definitions of success had ranged from coming off the operating table alive to surviving several years. DeVries himself would not have been satisfied with merely getting his patient off the table. "You can do that with a cadaver," he said. He had hoped to make Clark well enough to go home. Reiterating that the main goal was therapy, DeVries said that if Barney Clark had no regrets, then the procedure was a success. Social worker Peg Miller added that Mrs. Clark regarded the experiment as a "partial success," and Jarvik said that from the researchers' standpoint, it would have been "impossible" not to learn something. But, like DeVries, he felt that for the procedure to be called a success, "the patient must say it was worth it."

EXPERIMENTAL VOLUNTEERS

Regarding informed consent, Dr. Margery W. Shaw noted that Barney Clark had first seen the heart team's animal subjects in October of 1982 and then returned to his home in Seattle to think about the implant for more than a month. So he gave his consent freely, she said, without the coercive atmosphere of a hospital environment.

"Not necessarily," said DeVries immediately. "Disease is coercive." He then opened a whole new subject by disclosing that several healthy people have volunteered to sacrifice themselves to medical research by having artificial hearts implanted. One was a sixty-year–old woman who had finished raising her family, and the others were convicts on death row, who suggested that the machine could simply be turned off when it was time for them to be executed. All were turned down on the grounds that they didn't fit the criteria for patient selection. "I begged the issue," DeVries admitted, "by letting the protocol protect me." The death row cases would turn the surgeon into an executioner, observed Capron and Peterson. "Maybe we could have somebody shoot the drive system," DeVries remarked dryly.

On a more serious note, Reiser described such volunteers as "an affront to dignity." Capron disagreed: "They just make us uncomfortable. We're actually not respecting the dignity of their choice." After World War II, he said, when it was disclosed that the U.S. government had used incarcerated persons in order to conduct malaria research, the American Medical Association urged that it stop, that it deny them this opportunity for "their own salvation or earning back of grace"—not to protect patients, but to avoid making criminals into heroes or increasing their chances of parole. "We have since moved largely away from prison experimentation," Capron noted, not because of any affront to dignity but because the quality of consent is in question. Finally, he said, many people would be uncomfortable with death-row artificial heart recipients for the same reason that they're uncomfortable with execution by injection—it would make the physician into an executioner.

But what about the healthy woman who volunteered? Jarvik wanted to know what conference participants thought about her. "We actually draft healthy people to go to war and let them give their lives for national security," he said, adding that society even honors them. Why should medical volunteers be regarded differently? Because there is no great, urgent need for them to sacrifice themselves, answered Cassell.

Such volunteers always come forward, according to Fox. For instance, a number of people have offered Stanford University their hearts for transplantation. The surgical team there was "staggered" by the idea, Fox reported, and at first assumed the volunteers were "the most disequilibrated persons in San Francisco." But is it valid to assume that altruism always covers deep psychological problems? For prisoners, Fox noted, the sacrifice may offer penance and absolution; others may see it as a way of infusing their lives with meaning. But the medical profession doesn't seem to know what to make of altruism. Perhaps the best example of this, Fox said, is the profession's reaction to living kidney donors. In a long study involving various hospitals, she and a colleague came across a phenomenon they labeled "the blank live-donor chart." "It was almost as if the medical team didn't know what to write down on their charts," Fox recalled, because a healthy person had let himself be "injured" by doctors to help the "real" patient. And this is a violation of the admonition to "do no harm." Finally, she noted, physicians' conflicts over what they do to patients are revealed by the very words they choose to describe their work: calling surgical incisions "wounds," for instance.

INFORMED CONSENT

From here, the discussion shifted to the medical team's method of obtaining informed consent. Dr. Ross Woolley, a member of the Utah IRB who had more or less joined the heart team to monitor ethical problems, asked conference participants how the problem of the consent form ought to be handled. Barney Clark signed an eleven-page form, and several members of the audience admitted that they had trouble reading through it. Jonsen admitted that he fell asleep trying, but he also suggested that had the Department of Health and Human Services devised the form, it would have gone on for 140 pages. Observing that the riskier the experiment, the longer such documents tend to become, Woolley said, "Perhaps we've reached the point of logical absurdity."

No sick person should be expected to plow through an eleven-page consent form, according to Cassell. Rather, a family member or someone else close to the patient ought to read the document and tell the patient the problems, the benefits, and the past experiences. Then the family should talk; the patient could give his consent orally; and a relative could sign for him.

But there is a more basic question, one raised by Capron: "What is the consent form for?" Is it really meant to inform the patient or just to protect the hospital legally, to satisfy the institutional review board, the federal Food and Drug Administration (FDA), the university lawyers, and the insurance carriers that the patient has been told the facts? Maintaining that the form's main purpose is legal, Capron urged, "Don't confuse that piece of paper with the major means of education"—discussions and the subsequent building of trust between the patient and the medical team. If the institutional review board wants reassurance that those discussions are adequate, it should ask the medical team to sit down with board members and talk over the procedure as they would with the patient. Capron said he would prefer to sit on a board that conducted itself this way, one that trusted the doctor to keep his word and to talk to patients as he had to the board.

Others agreed with this assessment. Indeed, Cassell had said earlier that if Barney Clark had been surrounded by strangers he wouldn't have signed any consent form, no matter how complete; his consent was based on his trust of DeVries and the other members of the team and what they had told him in person. Reiser added that the gesture of asking for the patient's permission is also valuable, because it reassures him that the investigators respect his rights.

Another basic question, raised by Berenson, was whether there is any such thing as informed consent when the patient is agreeing to something that he has never experienced and even his doctors aren't sure what to expect. In such cases, the medical team must convey its own uncertainty to the patient, Capron said.

Perhaps the ideal consent form would be a treaty negotiated by doctor and patient, Jonsen suggested, instead of a formal document presented to the patient fait accompli. But DeVries thought that under the present protocol, such an arrangement would be impossible, because candidates for the artificial heart have life expectancies of only a month or so, not long enough to negotiate and get the resulting treaty approved by the IRB and the FDA. In addition, many candidates are too sick to negotiate. Barney Clark, for instance, was so ill that DeVries and his colleagues feared he might not survive the twenty-four hours that the IRB required must elapse between the first and second times he signed the consent form. However, DeVries conceded, people scheduled for coronary bypass could negotiate artificial heart agreements to protect themselves in case they could not be weaned from the heart-lung machine.

Capron then read aloud a passage from the autobiography of Philip Blaiberg, Dr. Christiaan Barnard's second heart transplant recipient. Blaiberg recalls the morning that a crestfallen Barnard told him of the death of Louis Washkansky, the first transplant patient. Barnard then asks Blaiberg to help him regain his confidence to fly again, to be, in essence, his next experimental plane. Blaiberg agrees at once, not only for his own sake, he says, but also for Barnard's. The surgeon replies, "a little more cheerfully now, 'Don't worry. Everything is going to be fine.'"

Barney Clark gave his consent under quite different circumstances, according to Woolley. But Clark's sentiments may not have been so different from Philip Blaiberg's. Woolley related that after DeVries and Clark read through the form together, Clark, wearing his reading glasses and propped up in bed with the form on his chest, looked up with a grin and said, "All I can say is, there'd be a lot of long faces around here if I backed out now." Woolley felt this comment meant that the document didn't matter: Clark had made his decision, and the form held no surprises. The real informing and the real consent had already taken place between Clark and the medical team. "What we saw," Woolley concluded, "was just a test sample."

PART TWO

Governmental, Sociological, and Legal Issues

The Role of the Federal Government in Artificial Organ Programs

GILBERT S. OMENN

INTRODUCTION

It is a pleasure to be invited to participate in this meeting. I think it is notable that those of you here in Utah are willing to review the many important aspects of the artificial heart program and to seek reactions and perspectives from those of us from other places.

I am well reestablished at the University of Washington, but I have been asked at this conference to draw upon my experiences in the federal government in order to broaden our discussions. I worked at the National Institutes of Health (NIH) 1967–1969 as a research associate; I was a White House fellow and assistant to the chairman of the Atomic Energy Commission 1973–1974; I returned as deputy to Dr. Frank Press, President Carter's Science and Technology advisor and director of the White House Office of Science and Technology Policy (OSTP) in 1977; and 1980–1981 I was an associate director of the Office of Management and Budget (OMB). I have served on the National Cancer Advisory Board; the National Heart, Lung and Blood Advisory Council; the National Council for Health Care Technology; the Joint Council on Agricultural Research; and the Interagency Committee on Recombinant DNA Activities. The OMB role involved responsibility for more than half of the federal budget, including all of the Departments of Health and Human Services, Education, Labor, the Veterans Administration, half of the Department of Agriculture, and two dozen other agencies. I have described some of the initiatives during my time in the OSTP elsewhere, including President Carter's goal to enhance basic research under the theme of "An Investment in the Nation's Future."[1] A more comprehensive review of the OSTP during the Carter years was published by Frank Press.[2]

THE GOVERNMENTAL ROLE IN
DEVELOPING BIOMEDICAL TECHNOLOGIES

I have been asked to talk about the role of the federal government in artificial heart implants. Let me begin by emphasizing the need for advances in biomedical research and medical care. All of you, clinicians and others, know that we are often frustrated by our inability to make precise diagnoses and by our inability to do much to change the course of many common illnesses, especially chronic diseases such as heart disease, arthritis and other degenerative disorders, mental diseases, and cancers. The needs and the challenges are tremendous. It is against that backdrop that we have to examine new proposals for preventive strategies, diagnostic maneuvers, and all kinds of therapies. It is not surprising that there is a great willingness to take risks, a great willingness on the part of the patients and their families, by society as a whole, and certainly by those charged with making progress, the physicians and scientists involved in medical research. There is also a considerable sense of optimism, undiluted by disappointments, that medical research and technologies applied to medicine will continue to yield advances in patient care. Sometimes lay people in this country have a better perspective than we physicians do, because we are so close to our frustrations and so aware that progress is more often incremental than dramatic. Many people remember when there was no treatment for pneumonia or when it was thought to be impossible to open the chest to perform a heart operation. I recall vividly the emotion with which President Carter recalled the fears of polio and the prohibitions on community swimming in the 1950s in Georgia, when he presented the Medal of Freedom to Jonas Salk in 1977.

I might add a personal note, confirmed in conversations last night with Dr. Bill DeVries. My mother's younger brother, who was fourteen years older than I, underwent closed heart mitral commissurotomy in Philadelphia when I was a youngster. None of us realized what a pioneer he was as a patient, but we certainly recognized the good results when he returned from the hospital no longer cyanotic and no longer short of breath. He himself was quite delighted with the results, but he had been stunned to learn upon recovering from surgery that, of the seven patients who had preceded him on Dr. Charles Bailey's schedule, not a single one had survived. He was Bailey's first survivor, I believe. That was 1952. Such surgery now seems antediluvian!

Government in our society is pervasive. It takes its strength from the interests and demands of the people. Governmental agencies are involved in all four stages of the process of bringing a new technology to the people. The first is the development of an idea or a concept, combined with animal research. The second is experimentation in humans. The third is the emergence of a new technology. It must stand up to scrutiny. What are the clinical indications? What are the medical, social, ethical, and economic ramifications? Finally, in the fourth stage, there is dissemination and incorporation of the new technology into regular medical care, which raises broad ethical, financial, and clinical questions.

The government, of course, has many parts. It is important to distinguish the roles of the executive branch, the Congress, and the courts. The executive branch is highly heterogeneous. In any agency there will be political appointees and career staff, including scientists. Agencies often have different constituencies and different priorities and operate under different statutory mandates. For our purposes, the agencies of greatest interest are the NIH research institutes and the Food and Drug Administration (FDA) bureaus regulating drugs and medical devices. Other executive activities may become important, as illustrated by the expansive role of the President's Commission for the Study of Ethical Problems in Medicine and Biomedical and Behavioral Research and by President Reagan's recent intervention to help a youngster and her family secure a donor for liver transplantation.

The Congress has quite a few roles, as well, with a plethora of committees and an estimated three hundred subcommittees. Through hearings, the congressional subcommittees can give visibility to problems and to proposed solutions. Through authorizing legislation, the Congress can mandate new responsibilities for executive branch agencies. And through appropriations and the language of the appropriations acts, the Congress can provide financial support and financial incentives for certain programs. The appropriations language may be so specific that the congressional intent determines the nature and location of certain programs or facilities.

Finally, in this increasingly litigious society, the imaginative and aggressive use of the legal process brings many matters newly in dispute to our courts for resolution. Several participants have indicated anxiety about the increasing role of litigation and the possibility of lawsuits. We face a growing problem.

Some people who aren't familiar with direct government decision-making have a notion that the government is an isolated monolithic structure that cannot be reached. But you must remember that the influence of outsiders on the government is tremendous. Very often a few people will be essentially in control of decisions, determining the direction, growth, public visibility, and public support for a particular program of interest. Perhaps the most impressive example of a private citizen who has influenced the development of the NIH is Mary Lasker.

Directing Biomedical Research

When we look at an overview of major diseases, what we might call the "killers and cripplers," there has been a clear mandate for the NIH to find ways to reduce the frequency and burden of illness. This mandate goes beyond developing basic knowledge. Thus, the NIH is distinctively different from the National Science Foundation. The NIH is, in large part, an applied science agency. Questions about the role, structures, and strategies of the NIH hinge on what kinds of activities are most likely to be productive in the short term and long term in reducing the burden of illness. There is considerable impatience about that agenda. The Congress, after all, has provided appropriations that make the budget of the NIH more than three times as large as the National Science Foundation. Most of the institutes have been named after diseases, and the two largest, by far, are the National Cancer Institute and the National Heart, Lung and Blood Institute.

In 1965 President Lyndon Johnson swooped down on the NIH campus in a helicopter and declared that he wanted "the secrets of the laboratory" unlocked and applied at the bedside in order to stem the tide of human illness. The biomedical research community has worked hard at developing applications, as well as basic knowledge. The strategy NIH has used has been a good one. Nevertheless, it is always under attack. Both past and present directors of NIH have put primary emphasis on basic research, seeking the underlying causes of disease processes in order to plan a rational attack on those diseases. In contrast, the artificial heart program is an example of a targeted development program.

It is not difficult to trace the history of objectives and program planning for the Artificial Heart Project. Over the past fifteen years, there have been at least five published reports. In October 1969, the Ad Hoc Task Force on Cardiac Replacement of the National Heart Institute published its report *Cardiac Replacement: Medical, Ethical, Psychological and Economic Implications.*[3] The 1973 report was entitled *The Totally Implantable Artificial Heart: Economic, Ethical, Legal, Medical, Psychiatric, and Social Implications.*[4] These two volumes covered much of the territory that we are addressing at this meeting, and more. There were smaller volumes published in 1977, 1980, and 1981.[5] Now a new committee is hard at work to bring the technical, clinical, ethical, and policy assessments up to date. The Working Group on Mechanical Circulatory Devices is chaired by Dr. Robert Van Citters of the University of Washington; one of the conference speakers, Dr. Albert Jonsen, is a member.

In the 1973 report, the Artificial Heart Assessment Panel stated, "We regard the potential advent of the totally implantable artificial heart as an earthshaking event."[6] That dramatic language was coupled with an impression that the advent was relatively imminent. Why has it required a decade to take the first step in humans, let alone move significantly closer to the widespread use of this technology?

The beginnings of the artificial heart program have been traced to the 1950s. Several investigators met at NIH to stimulate the development of a specific program in this area. Government programs typically begin in this fashion. As a result of that meeting, the NIH invited grant applications in the area of development of artificial and totally implantable hearts. Some proposals were received, but they were not funded. There was stiff competition for the research dollar, and there wasn't enough scientific content, nor was there sufficient bioengineering development. Within a year or so of the request for grant applications, the Advisory Council for the National Heart Institute became impatient. This was at the time that the White House was urging the National Aeronautics and Space Administration (NASA) to put a man on the moon. However appropriate or inappropriate was Dr. Chase Peterson's analogy of Barney Clark's operation to landing a man on the moon, there was a sense in the 1960s that directed programs like those of NASA could buy rapid progress in medical research. So the National Heart Institute council decided that research on the artificial heart should receive greater budget priority within the institute.

The Artificial Heart Panel was established in February 1964. Contracts were let to six firms in the aerospace industry to perform a systems analysis, and a report was published in 1966. However, an unexpected competitive approach arose in 1967 when Dr. Christiaan Barnard performed the first cardiac transplantation in man. Transplantation was suddenly in vogue. Over the next eighteen or twenty months, there were some 136 cardiac transplants; at least two patients survived one year.

Throughout seventeen years since 1966, there has been an artificial heart program at the National Heart, Lung and Blood Institute with a budget of approximately $10 million per year and with stable in-house management. It is quite revealing that I served on the National Heart, Lung and Blood Advisory Council for three years (1977–1980) without hearing about this program, so far as I can recall. Presumably, there was a constituency for keeping it going, but there was not enough of a push to bring it front and center to the main council and try to get substantially larger funding. During that period, the contract mechanism for funding was under attack; we were trying to put more monies into individual research grants and stimulate more basic research. Thus, there was not much receptivity in the late 1970s to invest more heavily in an industrial-style contract program.

It is clear that the outstanding advances here in Utah have brought the artificial heart program into a prominent position again. It will be very interesting to see how the National Heart Institute responds. The institute director, Dr. Claude Lenfant, has decided to go outside his bureaucracy and outside his own council to have a special panel reexamine the program and make recommendations, as noted above. Presumably, that panel also will take into account the recent resurgence of interest in cardiac transplantation. The use of cyclosporine seems to enhance greatly the success rate of the transplantation itself, but there are great difficulties in obtaining donors.

Despite a 30 percent reduction in mortality during the past ten or fifteen years, heart disease remains the number one killer. There is competition among totally implantable hearts, left ventricular assist devices, and cardiac transplants, not to mention all of the improving medical approaches. NIH can influence this competition both through its grants and contracts and through peer-review judgments and consensus-panel judgments.

The emphasis at NIH and across the federal government on basic research leaves open the question of how best to stimulate innovation, applications, and commercial developments. We know that basic research is necessary but not sufficient. In the Carter and Reagan administrations, and also in previous administrations, there has been a real effort to see what the government can do to stimulate innovation and early application of appropriate technologies in a variety of fields, including biomedicine.[7] Such efforts involve many policies other than research and development—patent policy, antitrust policy, tax policy, regulatory posture, and procurement practices, including payment for health services. It is clear that health care technologies drive an important sector of our overall economy. In addition, some of the largest corporations in this country are showing a substantial interest in what today is called biotechnology, stretching from genetic engineering to biomedical engineering and including mechanical devices.

Undertaking Experiments in Human Subjects

When one reaches the second stage, moving from experimental results in the laboratory and in lower animals to experimental studies in humans, it is clear that government has a role with a quite different array of activities. A variety of statutes place responsibility on governmental agencies to protect patients and to assure that certain procedures are followed. Institutional review boards (IRBs) and the informed consent requirements represent an evolving process for protecting human subjects and for doing so in universities and hospitals and other decentralized settings outside the government. The IRBs operate under authority delegated from the federal government, as recommended by the National Commission for the Protection of Human Subjects of Biomedical and Behavioral Research.

The FDA is required to consider the protection of human subjects in its approval of medical devices. There is no question that the FDA is extremely cautious in allowing the use of new drugs and devices. The FDA approach was influenced tremendously by the thalidomide tragedy in Europe. The FDA's delay and caution in approving that drug prevented an epidemic of birth defects in this country. It is not just over the artificial heart that the FDA is very cautious. The caution is reflected also in such a seemingly simple matter as approval of a radioimmunoassay kit to test for α-fetoprotein (AFP). This test is used to screen maternal serum to identify high-risk pregnancies for neural tube closure defects (spina bifida or anencephaly). The overriding, unresolved question in the AFP decision is the extent to which FDA should be involved in "regulating medical practice." I am sure some of you in this room have bristled at the kinds of questions the FDA staff raises when you submit information on an artificial heart device that meets your specifications and that has certain desired improvements over its predecessors or its competitors, such as not stimulating clotting. The FDA takes a lot of criticism, on the one hand, for overstretching and meddling in medical practice. On the other hand, the FDA is subjected to harsh criticism and legal challenges for not determining and regulating the indications for which a particular device or drug may be applied.

In the case of the totally implantable artificial heart, there have also been other agencies involved. In the 1973 report, one of the largest issues discussed was the potential radiation hazard and the question of disposal, after death, of the nuclear-powered mechanical heart in which the Atomic Energy Commission was involved. There was also some interest from the Department of Defense, NASA, and other agencies in the overall systems approach. The production of an

alternative heart is dramatic stuff; the excitement, the disappoint-
ment, and the drama were inherent in your experiments with Barney
Clark. I suspect that there will be more troughs and peaks, both technical and emotional, as this work goes forward.

Assessing Emerging Technologies

The third stage, the scrutiny and assessment of the emerging
technologies, may be the most difficult. Certainly we have yet to
find an efficient or even acceptable way to assess technology in medicine. In this country, we refuse to pay with our regular payment
mechanisms (Medicare, Medicaid, Blue Cross–Blue Shield, other
private insurers, or individuals) for any procedure or drug that is
called "experimental." However, when a bill for some new technique is approved for payment, then the federal government loses
control over its utilization, since it is no longer considered experimental. There is basically no control over which physicians can
apply it or for what indications. There is a tremendous need for systematic assessment of technologies that might be called "innovative" or "emerging"; they are in the big middle area between strictly
experimental work and established or approved technologies.

Some techniques are approved in the most haphazard way. When
one particular insurer or one particular Blue Cross plan, among all of
those around the country, pays, then others will say, "Well, if it's
paid for, we have to pay for it, too." There have been efforts for a
number of years to generate a more systematic and professional way
of performing assessments of emerging technologies. It is very awkward to conduct a meaningful assessment before the technology has
been applied to humans. Our present case of the artificial heart program is a good example. There are too many uncertainties—uncertainties about its efficacy, about the indications, about the costs, and
about potential complications. It is very hard for technology assessment to catch up while the technology is changing rapidly and the
uses and indications are being refined, often by off-the-cuff subjective judgments of physicians. Yet the need has been recognized, and
quite a few efforts have been launched.

The Office of Technology Assessment of the U.S. Congress has
supported and published a large series of assessments of health care
technologies. The NIH has set up an Office of Medical Applications
of Research and has held more than thirty "consensus-development
exercises," beginning with one on the use of mammography. A National Center for Health Care Technology was established within
the Public Health Service, with an outside council to direct its activities and with a charge both to stimulate and to evaluate medical

technology. Though appropriations for its work were very limited, the center sponsored several notable assessments and a rational priority-setting process. The American Medical Association and the American College of Physicians also have made significant contributions to the evaluation of new and existing technologies in medicine.

However, nearly all of these efforts are secondary analyses of existing information. Seldom are there systematic primary data-gathering studies using randomized clinical trials or other approaches. One of the limitations is the high cost of such trials, owed in part to what I believe is an inappropriate way of funding such evaluations. At present, the entire cost of clinical trials must come from the research budgets, and the patient-subject not surprisingly feels like a guinea pig. Clinical trials are organized to test alternative treatment or preventive strategies that are equivalently good or equivalently hazardous to the best of our knowledge. If that last statement is not true, then we face ethical barriers in designing and carrying out the study. I strongly believe that clinical care should be paid for by clinical care funds, under whatever payment source is available for each patient. Then the research funds would be reserved for the design of the protocol, the collection and processing of the data, and the extensive analysis and interpretation of the results. Clinical care and payment for the clinical care should be restricted to highly qualified providers and appropriate physician specialists who must agree in advance to full participation in the protocol and to the submission of required data. Some of these ideas have been presented previously.[8]

The National Center for Technology Assessment was abolished by the present administration. Now there is active consideration of a public and private consortium for technology assessment, which has been urged upon the National Institute of Medicine. An Institute of Medicine report, just released, recommends that such a consortium be established.[9] Its first task would be to set up and maintain an information clearinghouse, with a communications network among the various parties in the health manufacturing and pharmaceutical industries, in professional societies, in government agencies, among insurers, and among providers. The clearinghouse is intended to serve as a central repository of information on completed and ongoing assessments, to provide a forum for the parties with a stake in the development and validation of technologies, to reduce presumed redundancies in evaluation of specific technologies, and to facilitate dissemination of information on assessments. It is not yet clear whether all the parties will provide information, especially if the results do not serve their vested interests. This notion of a balanced private and public consortium seeks to overcome the suspicion that payers of medical care might be too cautious in welcoming new and costly technologies and that those with a financial stake in the development and commercialization of the technology might be too eager to promote its use.

If sufficient funding can be raised, the consortium would go on to perform secondary assessments, synthesizing results from reports and data generated by others; to stimulate primary assessments; to identify needs for assessments; to contribute to development and evaluation of criteria and methods for assessment; and to become involved in training and technical assistance.

There is another issue about the best measures for looking at the effectiveness of new technologies: randomized clinical trials, dependence on historical controls, or physician judgment. There will probably be different answers for different technologies at different stages. Another Institute of Medicine panel, chaired by Lincoln Moses of Stanford, is now at work on this problem.

Paying for New Technologies

I want to close with a few words about the management of these technologies, once they are agreed upon as efficacious and reasonably safe. Payment mechanisms in the United States are very awkward in dealing with the scaling up of these technologies. With coronary artery bypass surgery, for example, we are still paying at a rate that treats these operations as heroic, pioneering, and dangerous procedures. Yet Dr. Bill DeVries tells us that hardly anybody ever dies on the operating table any more, or at least so few die that it would be embarrassing to raise the question of whether they will need a backup procedure such as the artificial heart! The new prospective pricing mechanism for Medicare patients based on diagnosis-related groups (DRGS) is going to pay much higher (threefold to sixfold) prices for surgical care over medical care for patients who might be treated either medically or surgically. The profit margins for surgical care will be even greater, since the DRGS so far do not adjust for the rapidly declining length of stay now feasible for many surgical patients. For example, the price for bypass surgery is pegged to a median length of stay of 20.4 days at a time when the median length of stay for patients over sixty-five years of age is 11.8 days at the University of Washington Hospital.

An even bigger question than the price is, What are we buying? Do we have any way of getting adequate data to measure how effective a procedure is against the alternatives? Do we characterize the alternatives adequately? Do these questions belong to the business of government? Ideally, medical professionals should find ways to address these questions, but, for the most part, we do not. By default, then, these questions fall to government.

Many people believe that the least government is the best, except in cases where important social needs cannot be met through private mechanisms. For certain basic social programs, even the Reagan administration agrees that government must intervene to assist the "truly needy." We have decided, since the beginning of our country, that national security depends upon the federal government. We chose a federal initiative in 1957 for the space program. And we've decided that basic research is a primary responsibility of the federal government, because no private company has an adequate interest in supporting basic research whose results will be shared through publications and which may or may not have applications in the marketplace.

However, we generally believe that providing services and selling equipment is a function of the private sector. The private sector, as best as we can tell at the present time, has no orderly mechanism for identifying the relative merits of different modes of treatment for different patients. We can look at the controversies that have swirled for years over certain surgical and medical treatments. We realize that there needs to be some order brought out of all of this chaos and some general guidelines for how to proceed. In the present political climate, perhaps the government and the private sector can work together under a neutral aegis like the technology assessment consortium proposed by the Institute of Medicine.

It is apparent here in Utah, for example, that the team developing the totally implantable artificial heart had to become fully committed to this project and maintain that commitment for many years. It is impossible in such work to be dispassionate about the relative merits of the totally implanted heart, left ventricular assist devices, and cardiac transplantation, even for patients for whom medical therapy may no longer be considered effective. Harsh criticisms from some other quarters simply reflect the highly competitive situation among the surgical groups in this country. Added to the competitive nature of these technological developments are the complex institutional and financial arrangements of some of the principal players. Dr. Robert Jarvik, in particular, has been outspoken about the commercial aims and relatively short-term objectives of Kolff Medical. I am making no judgments about these relationships. I know that commercialization depends upon such firms. It is important that the relationship is openly acknowledged. It is commendable that key figures in the firm are participating in this meeting.

THE ROLE OF THE GOVERNMENT IN ETHICAL
PROBLEMS

An even more difficult subject to address than the definition of clinical indications and the levels of payment that would be appropriate is the federal government's role in the area of ethics. People have different values, and those values are not always sustained. People are challenged in their personal lives by events that they cannot anticipate. Sometimes they find that they must change their thinking (or what they thought they would have thought would apply to others) when it becomes necessary to apply those principles to themselves. We have had an extraordinary sequence of organized governmental activity on the ethical issues. Dr. Albert Jonsen has been a constant member in these activities. He served on the original National Commission for the Protection of Human Subjects. Then there was an interval during which there was an Ethics Advisory Board, established by the Department of Health, Education and Welfare. He served most recently on the President's Commission for the Study of Ethical Problems in Medicine and Biomedical and Behavioral Research, of which Professor Alexander Capron was executive director. Since the commission's mandate has expired, there is now a void in the government's focus on biomedical ethics, although outside research-oriented institutions like the Hastings Center and the Kennedy Institute at Georgetown University continue to grow, in part through governmental support of their projects.

I'd like to close by stressing the ethical issues because the inclusion of ordinary medical problems, access to medical care, and medical care decisions was an innovation in the mandate for the presidential commission.[10] This mandate reflected a desire to go beyond the review of research alone. We recognized that we permit ourselves as physicians, and society permits us, to use unvalidated technologies and to take chances with patients that no IRB would condone. Somehow we must bring the same high standards to ordinary medical care that we bring to research. At the same time, we must bring to research and development programs some of the "can-do" attitude that is so important in caring for patients. I believe that both goals are feasible, and I hope that this conference can stimulate such developments.

NOTES

1. G. S. Omenn, "Basic Research as an Investment in the Nation's Future," in *The Impact of Protein Chemistry on the Biomedical Sciences: An International Symposium to Honor Christian B. Anfinsen*, ed. A. N. Schechter, A. Dean, and R. F. Goldberger, pp. 7–19 (New York: Academic Press, 1983).

2. F. Press, "Science and Technology in the White House, 1977 to 1980," *Science* 211 (9 January 1981): 139–45; 211 (16 January 1981) 249–55.

3. Ad Hoc Task Force on Cardiac Replacement, *Cardiac Replacement: Medical, Ethical, Psychological and Economic Implications*, DHEW Publ. No. (NIH) 77-1240 (Washington, D.C.: Government Printing Office, 1969).

4. National Heart and Lung Institute, Artificial Heart Assessment Panel, *The Totally Implantable Artificial Heart: Economic, Ethical, Legal, Medical, Psychiatric, and Social Implications* (Washington, D.C.: U.S. Department of Health Education and Welfare, 1973).

5. *Report of the Artificial Heart Working Group* (Washington, D.C.: National Heart, Lung and Blood Institute Advisory Council, 1981).

6. National Heart and Lung Institute, Artificial Heart Assessment Panel, *The Totally Implantable Artificial Heart*, p. 87.

7. D. J. Prager and G. S. Omenn, "Research, Innovation, and University-Industry Linkages," *Science* 207 (25 January 1980): 379–84.

8. J. R. Ball and G. S. Omenn, "The Role of Health Technology Evaluation: A Policy Perspective," in *Health Care Technology Evaluation*, ed. J. Goldman, pp. 5–32 (New York: Springer-Verlag, 1979).

9. National Institute of Medicine, *Medical Technology Assessment: A Plan for a Private/Public Sector Consortium* (Washington, D.C.: National Academy of Sciences Press, 1983).

10. G. S. Omenn, "Presidential Commission on Bioethics Launched," *Bioethics Quarterly* 2 (1980): 76–83.

"It's the Same, but Different": A Sociological Perspective on the Case of the Utah Artificial Heart

RENÉE C. FOX

"It was the same, but different," they said. Implicitly and explicitly, this was a theme that was recurrently expressed in our conversations and interviews with members of the team who were involved in the implantation of the Utah artificial heart in Dr. Barney Clark, and in what preceded and followed it.

It was in June 1983 that Judith Swazey* and I spent a week at the University of Utah Medical Center, doing some firsthand field research in connection with the sociological study that we are conducting of the Utah heart implant. Our visit occurred several months after Barney Clark's death, while the team was still in an early phase of its postmortem stock taking. We were struck at that time by their dualistic perspective on what they had undertaken, experienced, and were still in the process of sorting out.

The team's "same-but-different" dualism had multiple origins and meanings. It reflected their shared ambivalence concerning whether, in the balance, what they had done was right and good. Their almost nostalgic remembrances of their recent Barney Clark past had an "it-was-the-best-of-times-and-the-worst-of-times" feeling about it.

Physicians, nurses, social workers, bioengineers, and members of the University of Utah's Institutional Review Board (IRB) and its Community Relations Department were all still deeply impressed with how "special" Barney Clark, his wife, and family were, humanly and morally, as well as biomedically. But, at the same time, they did not want to imply that they and the center were unaccustomed to caring for such sick patients or to competently mobilizing the complex medical science and high technology that it entailed. And they were concerned about giving the impression that they thought Dr. Clark was entitled to more of their attention, resources, esteem, and affection than so-called ordinary patients. (The intensive care unit nurses were particularly sensitive about these techni-

cal competence, distributive justice, and universalism-associated issues. As head nurse Linda Gianelli put it, they preferred to think of
Barney Clark as an "extraordinarily ordinary patient."]

Institutional pride and humility were also admixed in the team's
twofold outlook. The heart implant, they were convinced, was one
of the most important public events, and certainly the most newsworthy one, that had ever occurred at the University of Utah. It had
put Salt Lake City, the university, and the medical center on the
map, nationally and globally. Yet a number of team members were
uneasy about how rapidly and subtly pride can turn to hubris and
about the notoriety as well as the fame that being in the public limelight can bring in its wake.

Finally, the "same-but-different" orientation of the team also reflected their collective uncertainty about which aspects of their experiences connected with the artificial heart and Barney Clark were
concomitants of trail-blazing clinical medical research wherever it
occurs and which were particular, if not peculiar, to their own situation. The intricate blend of cosmopolitanism and localism, experience and youthfulness, sophistication and simplicity characteristic
of the team, and of the larger Salt Lake City, Utah, environment in
which it is embedded, contributed to this felt ambiguity.

In this paper I will identify and briefly discuss some of the sociomedical and cultural ways in which the Utah group's implantation
of an artificial heart in Dr. Barney B. Clark resembled other clinical
research endeavors and some of the ways in which it significantly
differed from them. My angle of vision derives from my continuous,
direct relationship as a field-working sociologist to the "experiment
perilous" world of medical research and therapeutic innovation, particularly dialysis, organ transplantation, and implantation, since the
early 1950s when I made a participant-observation–based study of
Ward F–Second, the male, metabolic research ward of Harvard Medical School's Peter Bent Brigham Hospital. The reason I chose this
topic is that my June visit to Utah persuaded me that clarifying its
"same-but-different" dilemmas is a critical part of the unresolved issues that the team faces as it looks back at Barney Clark while con-
templating a second heart implant.

LIKENESSES

To begin, How was the Utah artificial heart implant like other
clinical research endeavors involving human subjects? As is the case
with the first patient-subjects of all radical, experimental proce-

dures, Barney Clark, the recipient of the Utah heart, was a person rapidly moving to his inevitable death from a progressive, chronic disease condition for which there was no further established, effective medical or surgical treatment. The selection of a patient in this state for such a clinical trial was dictated by the uncodified but binding ethical assumption to which medical professionals adhere: namely, that a therapeutic innovation in the earliest stages of moving from the laboratory (or animal barn, as in this case) to the clinic, still fraught with all the uncertainty and risk that this animal-to-human phase of experimentation involves, should only be tried on individuals who are incurably ill, beyond conventional medical help, and close to death.

Barney Clark became what the members of the University of Utah Medical Center referred to as a very "special" patient. In their words, he was a "remarkable man" of great "courage," with a desire "to contribute to medical progress," and "to serve mankind." "He chose the unpredictable experiment over imminent death," they said, although he "knew he might have considerable anguish." Throughout the experiment (which lasted "for 112 days, . . . 2,688 hours, . . . [and] for 12,912,499 [heart] beats"), he displayed what team members described as "stamina, endurance, and persistence, . . . a sense of humor . . . and . . . ability to love (most of all, his wife and children)." Dr. and Mrs. Clark were regarded as "co-investigators with the research team in every sense of the word," and as part of the team members' professional and personal families. "Barney Clark is our hero . . . in this chapter of medical history," spokespersons for the team declared in their final tributes to him—"a pioneer to match these Western lands."[1]

There are striking similarities between the qualities that the Utah team eulogized in Barney Clark and how they related to him, and the way that the metabolic research group of the Peter Bent Brigham Hospital that I studied some thirty years ago felt about and acted toward their own patient-subjects on Ward F–Second. Even the language that they used to praise these patients and describe their relations with them is comparable to, and in many respects identical with, the vocabulary of the Utah team.[2]

The metabolic research group regarded its patients as "special." They were not only viewed as patients and research subjects but also as "colleagues" and "collaborators," whose "understanding" of the experiments in which they participated and "unfailing cooperation" in these studies made a professional as well as a personal contribution to the research. For the metabolic group, these patients were also "friends," who "at times seemed as close as one's immediate family." The physician-investigators were "impressed" and "inspired" by the "courage, . . . energy," and the dedicated sense of meaning and purposiveness of their patient-subjects. The belief and hope in the "perilous experiments" that patients displayed and their willingness to "suffer . . . stoically" for them in order to "help others in the future," if not themselves, "strengthened [the medical team's] determination," members said, to "go on" and "succeed" with the human research they had undertaken. The metabolic group expressed "admiration" for their "exceptional" patients and a sense of "indebtedness" and "gratitude" to them in various ways. "We celebrate our patients," they declared. They saw to it that their patients received "red-carpet treatment" in the hospital. They acknowledged the role that patients had played as "co-investigators" and "co-adventurers," by citing them in their professional publications. And they portrayed patients as "heroes" and "stars" in the news stories that they released to the press about the trail-blazing research for which the patients had served as subjects.

The observations that I recorded on Ward F–Second, in a Boston, Harvard milieu of the 1950s could have been written about Barney Clark and the medical team that cared for him and experimented on him in Salt Lake City, Utah, 1982. They are also applicable to the many other clinical research settings I have observed over the years. In fact, the "courage-to-fail" ethos of which these physician-patient relationships and values are a part was so characteristic of the organ transplantation and dialysis centers Judith Swazey and I collaboratively studied that it gave us the title for the book we wrote about them. *"The Courage to Fail,"* we explained in our preface, "epitomizes the bold, uncertain, and often dangerous adventure in which medical professionals and their patients are engaged":

> All have a high vested interest in the success of their endeavor. In their shared value system, a primary measure of success is the sheer survival of patients undergoing transplantation or dialysis. Beyond survival, it is hoped that these procedures may give patients an improved state of health that will enhance the quality of their lives. Success also means progress in medical knowledge and technique that may come from the collaborative research. For some of these physicians, and for some of their patients as well, professional and public recognition for their pioneering roles is an integral part of success. But the probability of failure in transplantation and dialysis is high. These therapeutic innovations are in a stage of development characterized by fundamental scientific and medical uncertain-

ties, and they are applied only to patients who are terminally ill with diseases not amenable to more conventional forms of treatment. In this context, the death of the patient is the archetype and pinnacle of failure for all concerned. Confronting this situation with courage is an ultimate value shared by physicians and patients. As they themselves recognize, the supreme form of courage that participation in transplantation and dialysis asks of them is "the courage to fail."[3]

In such drastic, path-making situations, there is usually a particular, senior physician–leader on the medical team who, in a charismatic, often tenacious, "don't-quit," indomitably optimistic, "we-shall-overcome" way, embodies this ideology and who exhorts and challenges his colleagues to live up to it. The Utah team has such a figure in Dr. Willem J. Kolff, pioneer over the past forty years in the field of artificial organs: beginning with his invention of the artificial kidney machine in Holland, during World War II, under Nazi occupation (a machine he built with his own hands, using artificial sausage skin for the cellophane tubing); continuing on to the development of the type of artificial heart that was used in Barney Clark; and extending beyond that to the work being done at present, at the Utah Institute for Biomedical Engineering, on an artificial arm and hand, artificial ear, and artificial blood vessels. "I tried four different machines and the last one became the first artificial kidney practical for clinical use," Dr. Kolff told the graduating class of 1983 at the University of Utah in his commencement address to them.

> Of the first 16 patients, 15 died. I then remembered the words of William, Prince of Orange, who said, "Even without hope you shall undertake, and even without success, you shall persevere." It was the 17th patient whose life was saved by the artificial kidney machine. . . .
>
> A number of doctors were opposed to the artificial kidney and wrote articles against it. I decided not to respond at all and to ignore it.
>
> I still have the same policy now that people tell us that the artificial heart has no future. . . .
>
> What have we learned from Dr. Barney Clark? In the first place, that the artificial heart inside the chest does not hurt. It does not cause any pain or discomfort. Second, the slight noise of the drive system did not disturb him. Third, the circulation could be adequately maintained. Finally, that this artificial heart indeed did fit inside the chest. Dr. Barney Clark has had more than his fair share of complications, most of them not at

all related to the artificial heart. In the periods that Dr. Clark felt well, when he could walk and go to the sun room, we know that his spirit was good, that he never lost his zeal for life, his considerable sense of humor, his desire to serve his fellowman, and his love for his wife and children. Therefore, all the qualities of the mind which make life worth living were preserved. . . . Of course, we are disappointed that Dr. Barney Clark did not go home. It is perhaps unfair to expect that the first patient with a permanent artificial heart would be a success, but you can be sure that "even without success, we shall persevere."[4]

Another major figure on the Utah team with a "courage-to-fail" perspective is Dr. William C. DeVries, the principal investigator of the clinical artificial heart program and the surgeon who implanted the artificial heart in Barney Clark. Dr. DeVries' sense of his relative youth (he was thirty-eight years old when he did the heart implant), his attitude of filial piety toward Dr. Kolff (for whom he began to work in the artificial organs laboratory when he was still a medical student), and his reluctance to assume a leadership role that is too moralistic and zealous in tone,[5] have made him more low-key and less public in his expression of these "you shall undertake, persevere, and succeed" values than Kolff. But inside the team (in the words of Donald B. Olsen, the doctor of veterinary medicine who is chief surgeon of the University of Utah Artificial Heart Research Laboratory), DeVries has been "the man of conviction" who risked himself and galvanized the group to implant the first artificial heart in a patient: "He believed sufficiently in our animal research data and survival times, and consistent abilities with the total artificial heart in sheep and calves, to gamble his professional future and integrity by implanting the artificial heart in man."[6]

Although DeVries welcomes the pause-for-reflection moratorium that the team is currently undergoing, he feels strongly that the endeavor must continue: "The project is bigger than we are. . . . I have no doubt about the device. . . . It works, and so I have to do it [a second implant]. Like the old Mormon song says, 'I must put my shoulder to the wheel and push along.'"[7] DeVries is actively engaged in trying to reunify the team around this conviction and "put new life" into the medical center's commitment to launching the next implant.

The kind of clinical research situation that the case of the artificial heart represents—with its front lines of life and death and medicine components and its competitive, achievement-oriented ardor both to win against great odds and to be recognized for being the first to attain such success—is a potential seedbed for the sorts of disputes over priority of invention, discovery, and development that so frequently occur among scientists.[8] It is not surprising, then, that the Utah medical center is confronted with a priority dispute over the "paternity" and the eponymy of the artificial heart implanted in Barney Clark.

The dispute centers around the claim made by Dr. Clifford A. Kwan-Gett that he has not received proper credit for his contribution to the model of the artificial heart used in Barney Clark—the Jarvik-7 that bears Dr. Robert K. Jarvik's name, rather than his own. Complicating the determination of who should be recognized and rewarded for making the most important scientific and technological contributions to this heart is the fact that, like other big, modern medical research projects, the heart's development spans many years and has entailed the participation of a large number of investigators from a wide array of disciplines in a team process with a complex, frequently changing division of labor. Within this framework, Kwan-Gett was intensively involved as a member of Kolff's group from 1967 to 1971, during which time he directed the animal studies and engineering research. He developed and laid the groundwork for a pneumatically powered artificial heart system and invented and designed the Kwan-Gett hearts upon which the Jarvik heart, with its superior fit, larger stroke volume, and multiple diaphragm design, was later based. (Jarvik, who initially worked with the Kolff team as a design engineer in 1971, returned to medical school in 1972 and after graduation in 1976 joined the artificial heart research group full-time.)

In his June 1983 commencement speech, with a touch of irony Dr. Kolff obliquely referred to the priority problem in the following way:

> This is the Jarvik type artificial heart such as was used in Dr. Barney Clark. . . . Dr. Tet Akutsu and I kept the first dog in the Western world alive with an artificial heart 26 years ago. That was in December 1957. . . . A great number (247) of different investigators have worked with me on various types of artificial hearts. I cannot possibly give credit to all my dedicated co-workers in this address. I am simply speaking of "we." When an investigator worked with one type of artificial heart, for ease of identification we gave it his name. Therefore, we have had Akutsu hearts, Nosé hearts, Wertzheimer hearts,

Donovan hearts, Kwan-Gett hearts and Jarvik hearts. The only thing we have not had is a Kolff heart.[9]

At this writing, the dispute has not been resolved but is being deliberated by a specially appointed university committee. However, it is interesting that a new, smaller artificial heart that was implanted for the first time 4 October 1983 in a calf was not named after a researcher, as many of its predecessors were. It was impersonally called "the Utah 100" heart, because it displaces 100 cc of blood. It would appear that partly as a consequence of the priority dispute it has experienced, the team is now eschewing eponyms.

The Jarvik-7 model of the artificial heart, a number of the physicians and bioengineers who contributed to its development, some of the calves on which it was first tried (Alfred Lord Tennyson and Ted E. Baer, for example),[10] the patient in whom it was implanted, his wife and children, key members of the complex medical team who surgically removed Barney Clark's own heart and replaced it with a mechanical one and who cared for him postoperatively, the University of Utah Medical Center and its various officers and administrators, the mountain-ringed valley of Salt Lake City—all became vividly familiar to the public through the more than 112 consecutive days of media attention that was focused upon them. Although in certain respects this media coverage was exceptional, the fact that one of the first human trials of a therapeutic innovation like the artificial heart proved so newsworthy is neither unexpected nor unprecedented. Health and illness, medical science, technology, and care are front-page feature article, major network news in our society. Increasingly, over the last two decades, they have become important foci—substantively and symbolically—of basic questions of value and belief with which we are currently grappling in our society. Even in the 1950s, when this was less the case than it is today, the so-called new wonder drugs, and new life-saving procedures that were being tried on Ward F–Second, and the stories of some of the patients who were experimental subjects were extensively and evocatively reported in newspapers and magazines. Barney Clark, then, was not unique in this regard. Rather, he was an especially large and beloved heroic figure in the American pantheon of tragic and triumphant research patient-celebrities who have been made famous by the media.

The fact that Barney Clark lost his human heart and that an artificial heart was substituted for it added extra dimensions of meaning and fascination to his case and increased the amount and prominence of coverage that the media accorded to it. In this respect, the kind of attention that it elicited and the way that it was treated by the press resembled the reporting of human heart transplants, particularly in their earlier phases. Along with the rational and factual scientific accounts of the artificial heart implant, certain magico-religious sentiments about the heart, akin to those that came to the surface in connection with cardiac transplants, also appeared. Judith Swazey and I found that "the development of cardiac transplantation . . . revealed that the heart is still widely viewed as the seat of the soul or spirit, the source and repository of love, courage, and the highest, most human emotions."[11] Such feelings and beliefs were apparent in the statements that the media carried about how glad Mrs. Clark was that her husband "still loved [her], even though he now had an artificial heart" and about how the Utah team felt that Barney Clark had "proved that courage and good humor and love of wife and children are sustained by an artificial heart."

There is something of the pathos of the Tin Man in *The Wizard of Oz* in this testimony, as well as magical thinking. For the American school children, who to this day continue to write to the University of Utah Medical Center in great numbers requesting photographs of Barney Clark, the convergence of high technology, one-giant-leap-for-mankind daring, and grandfatherly love that he personified seems to have made him an avuncular astronaut.

These, then, were some of the sociomedical ways in which the implantation of the Utah artificial heart was like other pioneering clinical research ventures. What were some of the differences?

DIFFERENCES

To begin with, the heart team's "special patient," Barney Clark, seems to have been even sicker and closer to death than the usual terminally ill patients who become the first subjects for a high-risk, experimental procedure, device, or drug. He was, in fact, sicker than the members of the Evaluation Committee discerned when they approved his selection as the recipient of the artificial heart. For, in addition to chronic, inoperable, end-stage, progressive, congestive heart failure (in its Class IV phase), it turned out that Dr. Clark also had severe chronic obstructive pulmonary disease that was partly independent of his heart condition. The fact that the selection criteria established by the Utah medical center stated that such an additional, "incapacitating medical illness" would disqualify a candidate for total artificial heart replacement and that the Evaluation Committee was explicitly charged with "the responsibility . . . to ensure the absence of other illnesses which would threaten the success of the artificial heart and render its implantation a costly but useless exercise" contributes to the inner controversy that the medical center and heart team are still working through, concerning whether or not Dr. Clark should have been chosen for the operation. Could Barney Clark's lung disease have been detected in advance? and Should it have eliminated him as a candidate? are not questions that a sociologist (albeit of medicine) has the competence to resolve or even to comment upon. But it may be of some relevance to note that, sociologically speaking, the individual selected to receive the artificial heart exemplified the "courage-to-fail" values of the Utah heart team. Directly and indirectly, this contributed to his eligibility in their eyes and strengthened his candidacy.

It was not only the biomedical condition of their patient-subject that distinguished the artificial heart team from other therapeutic innovators, but also certain aspects of the team's composition, organization, and functioning. On one level, the Utah group consisted of the whole array of professional persons who make up an advanced modern medical team based in a university hospital. But the team's own definition of its membership was more encompassing than is generally the case. As John Dwan described it: "The Utah artificial heart team extended from the patient and his family down through surgeons, Drs. William C. DeVries and Lyle Joyce, to University Vice President [for the Health Sciences] Chase N. Peterson, to the nurses, the therapists, the laboratory personnel, security, the patient selection committee, the social workers, the operating room staff, to practically every employee of the Utah Medical Center."[12] Dwan and his public relations staff were also considered to be part of the heart team. In effect, virtually the whole medical center was defined as the team, in a way that brought together modern conceptions of bureaucracy and traditional notions of extended kinship, that combined a strong sense of democracy and of hierarchy, and that placed Barney Clark and his family at the summit of the team. These attributes of the heart team's makeup are also basic principles and characteristics of Mormon organization.

In other regards, the team resembled the lonely and heroic situation in which pioneering innovators like Dr. Willem Kolff have historically worked. But the implantation of the artificial heart in Barney Clark was carried out by a surgical group that was unusually small and young when viewed within the time frame of the 1980s. The operation was conducted by thirty-eight–year–old Dr. William DeVries, Utah's chief thoracic and cardiovascular surgeon, and his associate and assistant, thirty-four–year–old Dr. Lyle Joyce (who had come directly to Utah only two years earlier, in 1980, after completing his residency in cardiac surgery and a Ph.D. at Minnesota). Only one house officer, Dr. Charles Berry, chief resident in surgery, assisted in the operating room. Doctor of veterinary medicine Donald B. Olsen, head surgeon of the University of Utah Artificial Heart Research Laboratory, was also present throughout the implant operation in the role of consultant. Dr. Robert K. Jarvik scrubbed in at the point when the artificial heart was inserted in Barney Clark and scrubbed out immediately thereafter. No other surgeons or surgeons-in-training were involved in the heart implant or in the postoperative care of Dr. Clark.[13] In fact, at the time that the implant took place, the center's Division of Cardio-Thoracic Surgery consisted only of Drs. DeVries and Joyce. The University of Utah had a two-year cardiothoracic surgery residency program that it ran jointly with the LDS Hospital in Salt Lake City and which included a rotation at the local Veterans Administration Hospital. However, out of the twenty-four–month training period that this entailed, the surgical residents spent only four months at the University of Utah Medical Center. They were not present at the center during the period of Dr. Clark's hospitalization. Furthermore, the chairmanship of the Department of Surgery was vacant.

The structure and dynamics of the Utah team differed markedly from other groups of therapeutic innovators in still other ways. Rather than centralizing the charismatic influence and authority it had generated through the scientific and symbolic import of its medical trail blazing—as pioneering clinical research groups are wont to do—and consolidating that charisma around the person and role of its physician-in-chief, the artificial heart team divided its charisma and distributed it among four of its members. The allocation and imagery of the team's charisma were also shaped by the media coverage that was accorded to the implantation of the artificial heart and its sequelae. Each of the four charismatic leader figures had his specialized place inside the team, and outside it in the sun of the media-conveyed public attention that the heart implant evoked:

- Willem Kolff, venerable and indomitable founding father, master inventor, and historic builder of artificial organs;
- William DeVries, young, modern, all-American, frontier surgeon of courageous conviction, with the physical and personality attributes of a Jimmy Stewart, Gary Cooper, Henry Fonda, and Abraham Lincoln rolled into one;
- Robert Jarvik, principal designer of "Barney Clark's heart"; boy-

ishly glamorous culture hero of bioengineering, in whom the values of the 1960s and of the 1980s seemed to be joined; artist and sculptor, as well as mechanic and physician, who took a long time to commit himself to medicine and to be admitted to medical school, and who, at age thirty-six, achieved Jarvik-7 fame and also business success as president and chief executive officer of Kolff Medical (a company that designs, develops, and produces artificial organs and related devices);
- Chase Peterson, chief medical spokesperson for the Utah artificial heart team, the medical center, and the university; intelligent and articulate, imaginative and candid public relations "star," whose at-once physicianly, teacherly, and pastoral persona conveyed a sense of medical and moral purposiveness, thoughtful responsibility, and team unity to the public.[14]

The development of these division of charisma patterns was given impetus by a phenomenon inside the heart team that was not publicly displayed. This was Dr. DeVries' strong disinclination to claim and control the charisma by organizing it around his status and role as surgeon-in-chief. Although he willingly assumed medical leadership of the team, he felt reluctant about taking on what he called its "moral" leadership. For him, such a moral role broached the domain of religion. As the head of a medical team located in Salt Lake City, Utah, where the Mormon population and Mormon church (The Church of Jesus Christ of Latter-day Saints) are centered, and as a Mormon himself, DeVries was concerned about acting too much like a church elder. In his view, engaging in such morally and spiritually tinged behavior on the basis of his office would be arrogant, particularly for a physician as young as he was. It might also contribute to Mormon–non-Mormon divisiveness on his team. And it could push him into a closer and deeper, personal and institutional relationship to Mormonism than he was ready for at the time of the artificial heart implant.

There are two additional respects in which the social system of the heart team and the way that it conducted itself distinguished it from comparable medical groups: the kind of ethical relationship that the team developed with the Institutional Review Board for Research with Human Subjects (IRB) of the medical center and the degree of familism that it exhibited in its relations with Barney (and his wife, Una Loy) Clark were both unusual. Along with a number of other factors (as in the case of the team's organizational and charisma patterns), the Mormon milieu in which the heart implant occurred latently affected both these two sets of differences.

The most strikingly divergent features of the Utah IRB crystallized around the role of Dr. Ross Woolley, the board's vice chairman, his conception of how the artificial heart implant ought to be ethically monitored, and the means that he used to do so. Dr. Woolley, an engineer with a Ph.D. in evaluation research and a faculty member of the Department of Family and Community Medicine of the University of Utah Medical School, became head of the special subcommittee that was formed to deal with the ethics of human experimentation issues in the case of the artificial heart. He brought to this role the strong conviction that the IRB not only had the responsibility to protect human research subjects and patients but also to protect the rights and principles of the institutions in which human experimentation and medical care take place. He formulated the term "protection of institutional integrity" to express what he regarded as the vital, institutional function of the IRB. Under his influence, the IRB attached greater conceptual and operational importance to this aspect of their obligations and activities than such boards generally do. Woolley and the IRB applied the notion of institutional integrity most vigorously to situations that involved attempts by the media to gain access to certain types of information about the center, especially those that pertained to the proceedings of the board itself and also to matters of so-called paycheck journalism. The chief paycheck journalism issues that the center felt it faced were questions about "the patient's rights to sell parts of his story, versus the institution's obligation to provide the essential elements to the public, versus the physician's rights to protect unpublished scientific data and patient confidentiality."[15]

Dr. Woolley implemented this view of the IRB and of its raison d'être by assuming a monitoring role that has few, if any, counterparts on other IRBs in the United States. By his own testimony, Woolley spent up to four hours a day in the intensive care unit where Barney Clark was hospitalized, throughout the entire period that Dr. Clark was a patient there. He made at least one daily visit to see Barney Clark until his death. He became one of Mrs. Clark's confidants and advisors. He read Dr. Clark's chart every day and studied his laboratory values. He made rounds with the heart team in the morning, often came back to the unit in the afternoon, and sometimes returned in the evening as well. He conducted extensive, ongoing, information-gathering discussions with a variety of team members. As he put it, he felt that it was his obligation to be very well-informed. The physician *cum* ethicist surveillance role that Woolley adopted took on some of the attributes of a medical and moral watchman. ("He is watching over us to make sure that we are living up to rules that exist in his head," commented one team member with a mixture of respect, irony, and indignation.) There was also an implicit priestly dimension to this role, which surfaced when Ross Woolley gave Barney Clark a Mormon blessing at the time of his death.

Woolley became what Chase Peterson has referred to as "our home-grown ethicist," partly because of the initiative of Dr. DeVries, who first invited him to "monitor the patient" and to act as a moral consultant. Only a few members of the team were aware of this invitation. Some felt uneasy about the scope and nature of what appeared to them to be Woolley's self-appointed activities. But the legitimacy of such a role and its advisability were not challenged by the heart team or the IRB until after Dr. Clark's death. Slowly and hesitantly, partly in response to comments from outside observers, the Utah group began to critically examine this "home-grown" role. Chase Peterson now concedes that it "was not well thought out." William DeVries admits that Woolley's role and behavior "overstepped bounds." And the IRB has decided that Dr. Woolley's in situ monitoring activities, inside the artificial heart team and in intimate contact with the patient-subject, are involvements that conflict with some of his IRB discernment and decision-making functions. Consequently, he has been asked to give up his IRB voting rights on questions that pertain to the artificial heart; and he has done so without rancor. As the team itself appears to recognize, there is something indigenous about the role that Ross Woolley came to play, the process by which it developed, and the fact that although it made some persons uncomfortable, it did not seem either unique or disturbingly aberrant to them. There is a sense in which the at-once democratic and authoritarian belief that "every worthy man is a priest" and the moral activism of the Mormon-infused Utah setting in which the implantation of the artificial heart in Barney Clark took place normalized the Woolley role. The Mormon context not only helped to shape this role, it also conditioned the responses of members of the heart team to it so that in the balance they regarded it as more familiar than dubiously strange.

The other singularizing sociological characteristic of the Utah team—what I have called its "familism"—also seems to have been influenced by the fact that the heart implant occurred in a Mormon milieu. I have already indicated that in other "experiment perilous" clinical research units I have observed, medical teams often become involved deeply enough with their patient-subjects to regard them like one of the family, as well as friends, colleagues, and coinvestigators. This was the case in the Utah group's way of thinking about and relating to Dr. and Mrs. Clark and their children. But the saliency of the heart team's sense of family, the ramifying extent to which it encompassed the Clarks, and some of its modes of expression all distinguished the Utah familism from comparable patterns in similar medical situations and groups.

Una Loy Clark was as central a figure to the heart team as her "special patient" husband. She was admiringly seen as the incarnation of an extraordinarily "courageous," "stalwart," "steadfast," "devoted," and "loving" woman, wife, and mother, who displayed great "endurance" and "vision" throughout all the days of "the experiment"; who shared her husband's "strong desire to serve and fulfill his mission," his "great hope," and his "considerable anguish"; and who sustained the heart team as well as Dr. Clark through her unvacillating "support to all." Una Loy Clark was the team's pioneering woman of virtue—their wifely, motherly, and grandmotherly "heroine."[16]

Even more striking was the way that some of the physician members of the heart team involved their own wives and children in firsthand contact and relations with Dr. and Mrs. Clark. At Christmastime, for example, they all feted the Clarks with a family party, complete with gift giving and Yuletide caroling. On New Year's Eve, at least one physician, his wife, and their several children paid a visit to the intensive care unit to see Dr. and Mrs. Clark and wish them a happy new year. Another physician's children visited the Clarks frequently enough to begin to think of them as an additional set of grandparents. There were also a number of times when a doctor's children made evening rounds with their father, and when one little boy slept overnight in a hospital room close to the intensive care unit so that he could spend some time with his physician-father who was on around-the-clock call for Barney Clark. By and large, the physicians saw nothing remarkable or problematic in this behavior or in the kinds of family connections they established with the Clarks. Rather, they considered such relations to be supportive and therapeutic for Barney and Una Loy Clark and also for themselves. In spite of the nurses', the social worker's, and the psychiatrist's concern about the disruptive impact of these extra persons and visits on the unit where Barney Clark was hospitalized and about the emotional demands that the team's family relations with the Clarks made upon them, these patterns persisted. The Mormon emphasis on the family as the basic unit of society, on the woman as the vital center of the family, on the desirability and importance of children, and on extended kinship and kinlike group solidarity seems to have shaped and reinforced these medical team attitudes and behaviors.

They would be unlikely to occur in this form, or to be permitted to continue if they did, in comparable hospital settings.

In the end, key members of the Utah team flew to the state of Washington to attend Dr. Clark's funeral, and the senior figure among them, Dr. Willem Kolff, delivered a eulogy to Barney and Una Loy Clark on his own and his colleagues' behalf. This was a consummate, ceremonial expression of the artificial heart group's familism. "Speaking for all of the members of our team," Dr. Kolff concluded, "administrators, doctors, nurses, engineers, technicians, physical therapists, dieticians—for all of us who were involved—we thank you, Una Loy, and your wonderful family for your trust and support and wish you Godspeed."[17]

THE "SAME-BUT-DIFFERENT" "COURAGE-TO-FAIL" ETHOS

Underlying the Utah artificial heart team's experimental venture, with its typical and peculiar features, was the "same-but-different," "courage-to-fail" philosophy that motivated and integrated it. The team's "courage-to-fail" outlook was articulated in an especially coherent, collectively self-aware, and thoughtful way. It was pervaded by what appeared to be a faith-filled, but more soberly responsible optimism than usual. This is the tone that Dr. Chase Peterson struck, for example, in his 18 December 1982 press statement: "It seemed to us," he said, "in the quiet of our consciences, that we were very deliberate, not over-enthusiastic, rushing into something that had a technological challenge to it. . . . We are overwhelmed with responsibility for Dr. Clark. . . . It is a milestone for him, a milestone for the human spirit." It was principally through Dr. Peterson that the team's ethos was put into words and communicated to the American public, along with detailed bulletins about Barney Clark's medical course. In his role as public spokesman for the team, particularly in the context of the daily televised briefings that he gave to the media people assembled in the hospital's cafeteria-based news center, Peterson was the key conceptualizer, imagist, and integrator of the team's shared perspective. Behind his representative role lay the year-long planning process in which he had involved the team in his capacity as university vice-president for health sciences, and what John Dwan has described as "the countless meetings, the repeated delineating of roles and responsibilities, the comparing of written scenarios, the round-table discussions, rehearsals, [and] barnstorming about contingencies" that this entailed.[18]

Below the surface of the team's version of the "courage-to-fail" *geist*, contributing to the unified way in which it was expressed and enlarging its meaning, are the values of Mormonism and the Mormon world view. To say this is not to imply that all or even most of the participants in the implantation of the artificial heart were Mormon. The Clark family, Chase Peterson, William DeVries, Ross Woolley, and Donald Olsen are all Mormons, for example, but Willem Kolff, Robert Jarvik, and Lyle Joyce are not. Nor was the heart team's nursing staff uniquely Mormon. Furthermore, the persons involved in the heart implant who are nominally Mormon vary greatly in the loyalty and fervor of their relationship to the Mormon religion and church and in their relative standing within it. They range from devout, actively involved, high-status lay priests, to alienated, so-called Jack Mormons and include various shades of "fence-sitting-middling,"[19] "lukewarm to cold" varieties of being Mormon that "do not fit into any neat categories."[20] It should not be supposed, either, that the tenets of the Mormon religion shaped the team's perspective and presentation in a totally conscious, deliberate, or doctrinaire way. In fact, as we shall see, the team is uniformly sensitive about any implication that "Mormon cultural or theologic principles," or that the Mormon church and "its life mold"[21] have shaped their undertaking. Mormon and non-Mormon team members alike consider overt references or claims to such influences to be "misleading," and potentially "damaging," regardless of who makes them.[22]

The fact remains, however, that Mormonism is a "gathering," a community, a distinctive culture and way of life, as well as a religion in the more conventional sense of the term. It pervades everything in the valley world of Salt Lake City, including the University of Utah, its medical center, and its heart team. The active commitment of the Utah group to developing a permanent artificial heart, its trail-blazing determination to implant the heart in a human patient, the personality attributes and qualities of moral character that the team sought in its first subject and that it found and extolled in Barney Clark, and its style of public reporting and accountability are all highly compatible with basic principles of Mormonism. The artificial heart implant dramatically exemplified, in a morality play–like way, fundamental principles of Mormonism: its pioneering, innovating history and perspective; its sense of manifest destiny; the at-once secular and spiritual importance it attaches to health and education; its conception of the human body as a tabernacle; the practical and this-worldly, but transcendental significance it accords to personal and collective improvement, accomplishment, mastery,

and progress, through vigorous human effort, animated by ratio-
nality, knowledge, and intelligence. These values and beliefs were
repeatedly expressed in the public briefings the team gave. Occasionally, particularly in Chase Peterson's statements, unobtrusive
reference was made to the explicitly religious framework into which
these values and beliefs fit: the Mormon theology of progressive self-
deification and divinization in an eternal growth process that spans
this life and the life that comes after it. ("We express our respect and
sympathy to Mrs. Clark and her children, and especially to Dr. Clark
who was—and I suspect is—a remarkable man, a pioneer to match
these Western lands," said Dr. Peterson in the press conference he
gave about Barney Clark's death.[23])

When confronted with this analysis of the relationship and fit
between Mormon values and beliefs and those on which the implantation of the artificial heart in Barney Clark rested, members of the
Utah team alleged that these principles were as American as they
were Mormon. "Mormon culture is uniquely American," Chase
Peterson affirmed. "While it may be more vigorously expressed in
1983 in the Mormon land than in Marin County, it is American!"[24]
This is indeed true; and herein lies what sociologist of religion
Thomas O'Dea has called "one of the great paradoxes of the Mormon experience":

> Despite the marked and genuine peculiarity of Mormonism . . .
> its typical American quality is no less real. . . . Mormonism [is]
> in many respects the most American of religions. . . . The
> Mormon group came closer to evolving an ethnic identity on
> this continent than did any other comparable group. Moreover,
> it was a genuine, locally and independently conceived, ethnic-
> ity, born and nurtured on this side of the water and not im-
> ported from abroad. Yet it also has been "an America in min-
> iature." The chief processes of American history have been
> repeated within the smaller context of the peculiar Mormon
> experience. . . . When we add to these historical processes the
> fact that in its values Mormonism offers an analogous spec-
> tacle of distinction and similarity, the strange combination of
> peculiarity and typicality stands out as the most striking Mor-
> mon characteristic.[25]

In this analysis of the Utah team's "same-but-different" profile,
the latent influence of Mormon culture and religion has emerged as
a significant factor. In largely implicit and unintended ways, Mormonism played a role in shaping the heart team's values, vocabulary,

and imagery; its conception of itself; its leadership and organization; and its relationships—to colleagues, to its special patient Barney Clark and his family, to the IRB, to the press, and to the American public. Mormonism in this sense added certain dimensions of meaning and mission to the implantation of the artificial heart in Barney Clark. It also helped to create some of the distinctive phenomena and problems that the heart team developed, such as its familism and its moral watchman role.

One of the earmarks of the Utah team is the exceptional capacity for self-examination and public scrutiny that it has shown. This group candor and openness notwithstanding, the team tends to react with great wariness and strong negative emotion to the suggestion that they were influenced by Mormonism (as I discovered when I shared this part of my analysis with them). The ways in which the team expresses this concern provide valuable further insights into its complex relationship to Mormonism.[26]

The team is convinced that making the Mormon factor manifest would "fragment" and "tear apart" their professional group and the working solidarity that it has achieved despite its potential Mormon–non-Mormon split and the ambivalence of some of its Mormon members toward their own religious tradition and church: "The team has kept [Mormonism] a nonissue. . . . We have worked hard to keep it separate. . . . We have not discussed it. It can only be divisive to get into it."

The team also seems to feel the need both to deny and to resist the controlling power of the Mormon community and church upon them and to take a stand against attempts on the part of Mormon institutions to interpret and use the artificial heart implant too imperialistically or evangelically:

> Can Mormon culture be presumed to be able to influence non-Mormons or the non-religious or atheists? Is Utah culture some sort of Chinese empire which absorbs or converts all those who come to conquer?

> It's a misuse of people to propagate these values. I don't think it's fair to claim that basic humanness—caring, cooperation, love, family—are exclusive to or even special to Mormons.

> In their way the [Mormon] church recognizes that the purposes of the [artificial heart] experiment were the same as their life mold. . . . The whole valley rallied around it and took it to heart. They saw it as divinely mandated because it fit their principles . . . and also because it put Salt Lake City on the

map. . . . People in the church look at Dr. Kolff in a very Mormon way, too. [In their view,] he left Leiden and Cleveland where he was unable to do his work, and he came out here to this beautiful wilderness, where he was left alone . . . unmolested . . . to develop and strengthen a delicate flower . . . his product of modern technology. The church sees Dr. Kolff as a kind of Brigham Young.

Members of the heart team disapprove of what they regard as such religiously self-aggrandizing conceptions. In addition, they worry about how this kind of religious reworking of the meaning of the artificial heart project and its transmission to milieus outside Salt Lake City and the Mormon world could adversely affect their scientific standing and their reputation for objectivity and fairmindedness: "It implies that [our] program is guided by religious influences." The fact that their first patient-subject, Barney Clark, was a Mormon makes them even more sensitively defensive about this issue. "Does it . . . assume . . . then [that we] favor certain patients partly on the basis of religion?" a team member asks.

The heart team is anxiously interested in being seen as scientific, secular, and both medically and entrepreneurially successful in an American way that goes beyond Salt Lake City, Utah, Mormonism, and the cultural and religious tradition of a "peculiar people." As one physician frankly stated, "Wherever I go in my travels, when I say that I come from Salt Lake, people say, 'Mormons.' . . . Salt Lake City is a very growing place. It is to its advantage to become more American and international as well. To the extent that people think the Mormon church controls things here, it's bad."

In the end, it could be said that the Utah artificial heart team's tacit struggle with Mormonism is a microexpression of a more general Mormon and American situation:

The Latter-day Saints have successfully created a Mormon community with its own values and social structure, although it is no longer a separate entity but is rather very much part, both geographically and sentimentally, of the larger secular society of the United States. Yet Mormonism retains much of its old peculiarity, and Mormondom remains in many respects a society in its own right and, as such, has been subject to a number of stresses and strains within its own structure. . . . The destruction of the semi-isolation of the last half of the nineteenth century, the growth of the gentile population in the intermountain West, the progress of modern thought, the dis-

persal of the Saints eastward—in short, the reintegration of
Mormondom into the parent culture and the accommodation
and compromises that it involved—raise once more . . . fundamental questions of "Why?" and "Whither?"[27]

The Utah heart team has entered a moratorium: a time of reflection that is moral and social, as well as medical and technological.
However self-searching its current mood may be, it is clear that the
team decisively intends to implant another artificial heart in another patient. When it is undertaken, the second implant, like the
first, will be done within the framework of Mormon-American faith
in "the reality of eternal progression," and belief that "improvement
[is] inevitable if man keeps working toward it."[28] In this view, one
does not hesitate for long on the edge of a frontier. Rather, in the
words of Brigham Young, by courageous and "faithful efforts," one
"earn[s] the right to take another step onward."[29] The Utah team's
implantation of an artificial heart in Barney Clark and its subsequent pause to reflect on itself constitute such "faithful efforts." The
next "step onward" will be their Artificial Heart Implant-2.

NOTES

*Judith P. Swazey, historian of science and medicine, is president of the
College of the Atlantic, Bar Harbor, Maine. Both Dr. Swazey and I are grate-
ful to the Human Qualities of Medicine Program of the James Picker Foundation for the funds that made this field research possible. I also wish to
thank Professor Willy De Craemer and Dr. Mary Ann Meyers of the University of Pennsylvania for their critical reading of this paper and helpful comments on it.

1. These quoted phrases used to describe Barney Clark are taken from
the interviews that Judith Swazey and I conducted with all the key members of the Utah artificial heart team (other than Dr. Willem J. Kolff, who
preferred not to be interviewed) and from the following three documents:
"Words Spoken by Dr. Willem J. Kolff at the Funeral Service for Dr. Barney
Clark," 29 March 1983; Willem J. Kolff, "Forty Years of Artificial Organs
and Beyond" (University of Utah Commencement Address, 11 June 1983);
Chase N. Peterson, "Terminal Events," news conference about Barney Clark's
death, 24 March 1983.
2. Renée C. Fox, *Experiment Perilous: Physicians and Patients Facing
the Unknown* (New York: Free Press, 1959); see especially pp. 85–109.
3. Renée C. Fox and Judith P. Swazey, *The Courage to Fail: A Social
View of Transplants and Dialysis*, rev. ed. (Chicago: University of Chicago
Press, 1978), pp. xvi–xvii.
4. Kolff, "Forty Years of Artificial Organs and Beyond."

5. The sociological reasons for Dr. DeVries' wariness about assuming this kind of moral leadership role will be discussed later in this paper.

6. Donald B. Olsen, as quoted in "Total Artificial Heart Development at U. of U." (University of Utah News Service release, 22 December 1982), p. 8.

7. William C. DeVries, interview with author, 14 October 1983.

Another phenomenon that the Utah team shared with other clinical research groups is the moratorium on artificial heart implants that has ensued since the death of Barney Clark. As Judith Swazey and I have written elsewhere, such "moratoriums have occurred repeatedly in the history of therapeutic innovations. Typically, a moratorium takes place when the uncertainties and risks of a new treatment become starkly apparent and the patient mortality seems unbearable or unjustifiable. Pressure for a moratorium can come from physician-investigators' own reactions to the situation, from their colleagues, from the institution in which they work, or from patients and their families. . . . A clinical moratorium . . . may last for weeks, months, or years" (*Courage to Fail*, p. 108). See "The Heart Transplant Moratorium" (chapter 5) in *Courage to Fail*, pp. 108–34, and also Judith P. Swazey and Renée C. Fox, "The Clinical Moratorium: A Case Study of Mitral Valve Surgery" in *Experimentation with Human Subjects*, ed. Paul A. Freund, pp. 315–57 (New York: George Braziller, 1970). We hope to write a detailed account of the Utah team's moratorium in a future paper.

8. See Robert K. Merton's classic essay "Priorities in Scientific Discovery," first published in *American Sociological Review*, 22 (December 1959): 635–69, and reprinted in Robert K. Merton, *The Sociology of Science*, ed. Norman W. Storer, pp. 286–324 (Chicago: University of Chicago Press, 1973).

9. Kolff, "Forty Years of Artificial Organs and Beyond."

10. The naming of the calves and sheep that have been recipients of artificial hearts is structured by an interesting set of norms and folkloric practices that have developed in the Utah artificial heart laboratory and barn.

The principal surgeon and investigator for a given implant is the person who has the right and privilege of naming the animal-recipient. The name is usually not given to the animal until at least twenty-four hours after the implant has occurred. Dr. Donald B. Olsen, who directs the animal work, attributes this custom to the fact that in the early days of the artificial heart program, there was great uncertainty concerning whether the animal into which a heart was implanted would survive even that long. Investigators say that they try to choose a name that "fits the animal's personality" or the surrounding circumstances under which the implant is done. For example, the name Fred was given to "an extremely ugly animal, with a wonderful personality"; and a female calf who received a heart implant on Columbus Day was named Niña after one of Columbus's ships. More often than not, the names chosen are humorous, such as Ali Baa Baa for a sheep. The names in which the investigators seem to take the greatest pleasure are those that make some sort of self-mockingly romantic or ironic commentary on the meaning of their experimental work, such as Alfred Lord Tennyson, Magic, or in the case of twin calves, Charles and Diana. In the last instance, the fact that "Diana gave her heart to Charles" in an experimental heart transplant added a dimension of gallows humor to the significance of their interconnected names.

The observations that I have made in other laboratories over the years lead me to believe that these and other social patterns and cultural traditions that have grown up in the Utah artificial heart group are not idiosyncratic. There is rich sociology of science content in such laboratory behavior that has been largely overlooked by social scientists.

11. Fox and Swazey, *Courage to Fail*, p. 29.

12. John Dwan, "The Public Relations of an Artificial Heart Implant," American Association of Medical Colleges News & Comment, typescript.

13. In addition, a fourth-year medical student, Patricia McNabb, was present, along with anesthetists and surgical nurses in their vital operating room roles.

14. In June 1983, after the implantation of the artificial heart in Barney Clark and his subsequent death, Chase Peterson became president of the University of Utah.

15. Dwan, "The Public Relations of an Artificial Heart Implant."

16. The quoted statements about Una Loy Clark are drawn from our interviews with members of the Utah artificial heart team and from the various University of Utah documents previously cited.

17. "Words Spoken by Dr. Willem J. Kolff at the Funeral Services for Dr. Barney Clark."

18. Dwan, "The Public Relations of an Artificial Heart Implant."

19. This is the way one of the members of the Utah team described his relationship to Mormonism.

20. Thomas F. O'Dea, *The Mormons* (Chicago: University of Chicago Press, 1957), pp. 184–85.

21. The quoted phrases in this sentence are excerpted from interviews with two different Mormon members of the artificial heart team.

22. These quotes come from an interview with a non-Mormon member of the Utah team.

23. Peterson, "Terminal Events."

24. This statement was part of Chase Peterson's public response to the version of this paper presented at the conference of the artificial heart implant team in Alta, Utah, 13–15 October 1983.

25. O'Dea, *The Mormons*, pp. 117–18.

26. The following quotations from members of the artificial heart team come from both public and private discussions that I had with them concerning their reactions to the analysis of the influence of Mormonism on the artificial heart implant. That analysis was presented at the 13–15 October 1983 conference in Alta, Utah, where they were all gathered.

27. O'Dea, *The Mormons*, pp. 222, 258.

28. Mary Ann Meyers, "Gates Ajar: Death in Mormon Thought and Practice," in *Death in America*, ed. David E. Stannard, p. 113 (Philadelphia: University of Pennsylvania Press, 1975).

29. Brigham Young, as quoted in Meyers, "Gates Ajar," p. 114.

The Role of the Lawyer and Legal Advice in the Artificial Heart Program

ALEXANDER MORGAN CAPRON

The first implantation of a permanent artificial heart in a human being and the implantations that seem likely to follow in the next several years raise a host of important issues of public policy. These issues will be resolved, for good or ill, through the various parts of our legal system, including the courts, Congress, and the executive agencies, such as the Health Care Financing Administration. But the search for policies that are both rational and ethically justifiable is not advanced by labeling these issues as "legal," although it is doubt-less true that the consideration of an issue by a particular lawmaking institution can shape that issue in subtle and sometimes unnoticed ways. Nonetheless, it seems to me that the hardest questions—those about when it becomes justifiable in the process of developing such a device as an artificial heart to use it in human subjects and about how, once we pass the few patients like Dr. Barney Clark with severe cardiomyopathy, treatment decisions are going to be made about the 250,000 Americans who die of myocardial infarctions each year in hospitals and might thus be candidates for an artificial heart—are not in any narrow sense lawyers' questions.

Rather than elaborate on these larger issues, which are really matters of common concern to all of us participating in this confer-ence, I have chosen to focus on a few particular issues that have a decided legal component. In doing so, I hope to fulfill the charge that Dr. Margery Shaw gave me, not to spin out grand theories but to serve, in effect, as a consultant on the particular case before us here.

WHAT ISSUES ARE LEGAL?

To begin, I must emphasize the tentative nature of my remarks. Even after twenty-four hours of immersion in the Utah scene, one cannot know enough to reach many judgments about what went on here, and consequently, what the legal, or other, issues are. Further-more, as I told the meeting's organizers at the outset, I have mis-givings about structuring a meeting around disciplines. I doubt that subjects like the artificial heart are best analyzed in terms of legal issues, social issues, economic issues, and medical issues. Rather, they should be broken down by issues of substance, such as the selec-tion of subjects, the competence of subjects, commercial/industrial-university relations, and equity in the use of resources. On each of these topics contributions can be made by people from medicine, from science, from law, from sociology, and from ethics.

Nevertheless, once the format had been selected, my interest was piqued by the view, originally expressed to me by Marge Shaw and confirmed by a number of people who were closely involved in the first implant, that there had been little, if any, legal input in the artificial heart program. At the very least my fraternal instincts were offended. What, no lawyers? After the indignation wore off, I recon-sidered and found myself thinking, "But that's not surprising. There weren't any distinctly legal issues anyway, so why should any law-yers be centrally involved?"

Suppose then, that the legal input had been limited, as several people have told me, to routine review by the hospital's attorney and the university counsel? What issues might one list that a detailed legal analysis would turn up? First, of course, would be the ques-tions of medical malpractice. Yet, one of the striking things about medical research is how very few suits have ever been brought against researchers. Of course, in this particular area, the suit brought by the widow of Mr. Karp against Dr. Denton Cooley stands out as one of those few examples, but they are few and far between.[1] Unlike the epidemic of medical malpractice cases, we have not had an epidemic of suits for "malresearch."

Similarly, the other legal issues that the artificial heart case pre-sented hardly seemed of major significance, at least in the context of the present discussions. For example, the regulatory status of the de-vice is of importance to the implant team and involved extensive ne-gotiations between the Food and Drug Administration (FDA) and the University of Utah, without raising theoretical conundrums. Like-wise, lawyers might be interested in the control over the proprietary interests involved, which is a matter of contractual negotiations be-tween the University of Utah and Kolff Medical. Some fascinating legal intricacies might arise, but they are of a technical nature that would not be of general concern to us.

Anyone studying the artificial heart case must also be struck by the complex interaction of the implant team with the university's institutional review board (IRB). Yet, again, the most fascinating aspects are not the legal ones. The law is embodied here in the regulations of the Department of Health and Human Services and of the FDA that require prior IRB approval, according to certain standards and procedures. But the unusual aspects go well beyond the rules to the psychology and sociology of what occurred. On the legal side, IRB approval was given in this case by a duly constituted group, which was even represented during the months of Dr. Clark's care by a representative or monitor—a step into the actual implementation of the protocol that is much more than has existed in most research studies. So there doesn't seem to be a legal issue there. Even the definition of death, an issue that has held the attention of physicians, lawyers, and legislators the last fifteen years, did not seem to be a big matter here. Under Utah law, a body supported by an artificial heart and by artificial pulmonary support would be recognized as dead after all functions of the brain had ceased.

Therefore, the most important issues raised by the artificial heart—the selection of subjects and the process by which patients become involved in this project (which might come under the heading of "informed consent")—are not distinctively legal issues. The law may establish requirements or standards vis-à-vis such issues, but it does so in its role as a means of implementing social decisions, not on the basis of unique legal values. The law does have a normative content, but in the context of the selection of subjects, any number of value choices could be made that the legal system would be capable of implementing, depending upon the mode of operation desired. We need only think, as Guido Calabresi and Phil Bobbitt pointed out in their book on tragic choices, about the raising of an army.[2] Within the last fifteen years we have adopted, as a social view, a series of attitudes about the way the armed forces should be raised. First, we opted for considerations of social merit or usefulness, which were embodied in a system of draft deferments for men of selected status or occupations. Then when society became uncomfortable with that, we moved to a system that relied on randomness, the draft lottery. And then, when that seemed to produce unnecessary or unacceptable results, we turned to the marketplace and adopted the system of a volunteer army in which people are paid for their services as an alternative to other forms of employment. Thus, the law is capable of adapting; it can express different value preferences in each context. Similarly, in the area of catastrophic diseases, legal rules could be promulgated based on age cut-offs, financial criteria, a first come–first served arrangement, or medical criteria. Each of these could be incorporated through different legal standards, depending upon the formulator's value preferences and objectives.

The law does, of course, place certain constraints on some choices. Certain societal values take the form of constitutional provisions or statutory requirements that may restrict other programmatic choices. But the force of these societal values is not that they come from the law as such. Rather, these are societal values that have become embodied in the law, which, therefore, places limitations on what a research scientist or an institution could adopt by way of a policy. Even an issue like informed consent—which has, after all, been created by judges and, to a lesser extent, by legislators—is really an attempt to embody societal values about self-determination and the protection of well-being. The law can embroider on the details of informed consent, that is to say, whether the standard should be the information that physicians usually disclose or the information that a reasonable patient would want or need, but it is merely attempting to translate a social consensus, whether through legislation or judicial decision.

FRAMEWORK OF ANALYSIS

Nonetheless, I believe there are several other issues that, although perhaps no more distinctively legal than those mentioned above, have traditional legal features and do not seem to have been addressed by lawyers in the process of planning for this implant project. I continue to think that the "legalness" of these issues is only one of their aspects rather than to define them exclusively by a distinctive set of values and norms; other people who come from the fields of biomedical science, economics, or ethics may have other approaches to these issues. In other words, the task I see the law performing here is to suggest solutions in anticipation of the occurrence of a problem that is still theoretical as well as to provide practical solutions to problems that have actually arisen, rather than imposing a particular set of views or values. As Jay Katz and I explored in a book we wrote a dozen years ago,[3] the specific content of a problem, as well as who should attempt to solve it and in what way, will vary, depending upon the stage of decision-making. Drawing on that work, my stages here—the formulation of a policy, the implementation of that policy, and the review of its consequences—are somewhat different from the ones that Dr. Gilbert Omenn mentioned earlier because I am addressing a somewhat different issue.[4]

To take one example, it seems to me that IRBs, which exist at the point of implementation, are poorly situated to reach overall judgments about resource allocation. To rely on them for this is really inappropriate, just as it would also be inappropriate if the IRB were to take on as its major role the protection of the research institution rather than the protection of subjects. Others may disagree with this view. (John Bunker, for example, has expressed a very expansive view of the role of IRBs.) My concern is that, of late, society has placed excessive reliance on local committees in lieu of grappling with the difficult issues and formulating policies adequately at an earlier stage in the decision-making process. The IRB is more suited, by membership and tradition, to *implement* policies aimed at ensuring the suitability and safety of research.

Instead of relying on an IRB to reach the "macro" decisions for which it is ill-suited, we should take on these sorts of issues on a broader basis than a single institution's committee and at an earlier point in policy formulation. An example of one such effort is the report *Securing Access to Health Care*,[5] prepared by the President's Commission for the Study of Ethical Problems in Medicine and Biomedical and Behavioral Research, which sets forth a framework for resolving those kinds of issues on a level that doesn't just pass them along unresolved to a local committee. Therefore, the framework for my remarks is twofold: that the law is a means to an end and that it should adjust itself to the appropriate stage in the decision-making process.

THREE LEGAL ISSUES

For the remainder of this discussion, I would like to focus on three issues that have particular legal content: first, the termination of treatment, or the issue of euthanasia; second, the issue of surrogate decision-making for an incapacitated patient; and third, the issue of privacy.

Termination of Treatment

The hope for Barney Clark's artificial heart was that it would restore cardiac functioning, allow a more normal existence, and relieve the pain of a heart in collapse. Chase Peterson was quoted as saying that he thought Barney Clark either would die one to two days after the operation or would go home in ten days—in other words, the medical team did not foresee a middle ground as likely. It was unfortunate that this first attempt ended in that middle ground, especially because it resulted from a number of particular setbacks, such as seizures, valve fracture, and pneumothorax. But the actual middle ground was fortunate in avoiding what apparently came to be seen as the worst possible situation—having to cease treatment while not only the heart but some functions of the brain were intact. As I understand it, on 23 March within a matter of twelve hours or so, Dr. Clark, like the proverbial one-horse shay, simply fell apart and died of circulatory collapse, secondary to multiorgan system failure. What if it had not been like that, however? Specifically, what if Dr. Clark had simply become tired of living with an artificial heart and wanted to disconnect the apparatus, or alternatively, what if he had lapsed into a coma but still retained some brain function and the treatment team decided further efforts would be futile? I'd like to examine these two alternative outcomes that could have happened but didn't.

Usually, in situations of the first type, in which choices about treatment are being made by the patient, the choices are seen as morally less problematic than in the second situation in which choices must be made by one or more people on behalf of an incompetent patient. But in these two hypothetical situations it would appear that the reverse would be the case. At least from the personal viewpoint, the first situation of a direct choice to die would probably be a more difficult situation for the patient, family, and health care team to encounter. Some of the reasons for that are not specifically legal. For example, the way in which Dr. Clark had been cast into the role of a brave frontiersman would have made it extremely difficult, existentially, for him to choose death as the preferable alternative to continued treatment.

The legal setting for these decisions involves two connected issues—the contractual arrangements and expectations among all parties and the limits set by the criminal law. Anyone attempting to analyze this situation from the outside is on somewhat shaky ground because Dr. William DeVries, the nurses, the members of the selection committee, and all the others involved had a much more complex interaction and relationship with Barney Clark than can be gathered from a few pieces of paper, and I am sure that it is not adequately or fully encapsulated in the language of the special consent form. But with that caveat, since that is all I have, it seems to me that, in addition to its awkward phrasing and redundancy, the consent form contains some very strange information about treatment termination. Specifically, paragraph 16, which is quite brief, states: "I understand I am free at any time to withdraw my consent to participate in this experimental project, recognizing that the exercise of such an option after the artificial heart is in place may result in my death."

That language strikes me as very odd on several counts. First, in the first clause, the legally correct language of "withdraw . . . consent" is used. Isn't what is really meant is withdrawing from the project itself? The next phrase ends with the language "may result in my death." What can that mean? That I, Barney Clark, retain the heart, but withdraw from the project; that is to say, I'll no longer be in the experiment, but there is a therapeutic version of this heart as well as the experimental version? Or, alternatively, that although I will withdraw my consent, the physicians won't listen to me anyway, and they will go on treating me and leave the heart in? Or, finally, can it mean—miraculously—that I can live without a heart?

Basically, it seems as though one of the fundamental issues with the artificial heart—whether the patient can turn it off or have it turned off and die—was treated in a very unclear and evasive way. The consent form not only failed to confront this legal and emotional issue but actually sowed seeds of further confusion. My belief that there may be some accuracy to this interpretation is reinforced by the following passage in Lawrence Altman's 12 April 1983 *New York Times* account of an interview with Dr. DeVries. In this he wrote:

> Dr. Kolff had caused a stir, when in response to reporters' questions, he described how an artificial heart recipient could end the experiment by suicide: a key in the powering device could be turned or scissors could be used to cut the hoses that carry the compressed air that keeps the heart beating. Dr. Clark learned of these comments and called Dr. Kolff "the man with the scissors."
>
> About three weeks after the heart was implanted, Dr. Kolff walked into Dr. Clark's room while the artificial heart recipient and Dr. DeVries were talking. As Dr. Kolff walked over to inspect the air pump, Dr. Clark nervously asked what they were doing. Dr. DeVries explained and told the retired dentist not to worry. As Dr. Kolff walked away, Dr. Clark relaxed.
>
> Then Dr. Kolff walked back toward the power system. "Barney got nervous again, and his eyes started popping," Dr. DeVries said. "Then Dr. Clark said, 'Don't quit, don't quit.' He was scared for the first time that someone was going to do that to him, and it took me almost a night to explain that we were not stopping."

This description of Dr. Clark's state of mind certainly indicates that it is problematic to believe that everyone involved was comfortable with "the key."

What about a direct request from Dr. Clark? How would that have been evaluated? Again, Lawrence Altman's interview provides us with some information about that. He describes the period in which Dr. Clark had nosebleeds, and it was very difficult for the patient to breathe because there was gauze in his nose and he tended to gag:

> Many such patients have complained without truly meaning their words that they preferred death to treatment. Dr. Clark did, too, according to Dr. DeVries, who recalled: "When Barney was very confused and disoriented and his nose was packed to stop the bleeding, he asked me and the nurses, perhaps five times, 'Why don't you let me die?'"
>
> Did Dr. Clark really mean it? [That was a question from Dr. Altman.] "That's what we all asked," Dr. DeVries said.
>
> Doctors have their ways of assessing such situations. One way is to observe if a patient continues to express such wishes over a long period. Another is to observe a patient's behavior. Some become aggressive and hostile to the point that they no longer cooperate.
>
> "Barney never got that way—he was perfectly cooperative in every single thing we did," Dr. DeVries said, adding that Dr. Clark did not repeat the sentiment.

It seems to me that this was a form of ad hoc decision-making about the competency issue and at what point one would listen to Dr. Clark. Again, I have to base my analysis on the written statement—which I gather the IRB and the FDA both approved—that details the group of patients with whom the device could be used. This protocol does not contain an evaluation of the policy to determine when to respect and when not to respect a patient's stated wish that the patient wants to withdraw from the experiment. It is stated in the consent form: "I am free at any time to withdraw my consent." But clearly that was not taken to be a literal statement, although one does not know the standards that were used to decide when to treat a patient's wishes literally and when to disregard them. This is unfortunate in light of the emphasis (as noted over the past dozen or so years by a series of reports by government panels examining the artificial heart experiment) on the need to avoid ad hoc decision-making and to establish clear policies that will guide the case-by-case implementation.[6]

The question of treatment termination can be taken one step further. How would the university have felt had Barney Clark requested a termination and had met whatever criteria for a competent decision had been established or were established at that time? I must rely on my rapporteurs in the University of Utah administration. They have told me that although the consent forms had gone through the hospital's lawyers and the university's outside counsel, the forms received only perfunctory review (which had addressed, for example, the issue of not promising compensation for any research injuries). The lawyers had not discussed the criminal law aspects of treatment termination. Nonetheless, when questioned during press conferences about Dr. Clark's ability to withdraw from treatment, Dr. Peterson agreed that such an act would be suicide, and he opined that the university might incur civil or criminal liability for acquiescing in such a request. Although I disagree with that conclusion as a substantive matter of law, the important point for the moment is that Dr. Peterson's statement indicated a wholly different view of the acceptability of treatment termination than was nominally described in the consent form. I wonder what Dr. Clark thought about this if he heard it on the TV or radio or read it in the papers. Moreover, it does seem remarkable, with all the attention paid to certain legal matters by the IRB and FDA, that this important issue was not addressed in advance, leaving policy to emerge in response to the reporters' questions.

Surrogate Decision-making

It is difficult to see why the issue of surrogate decisions wasn't explicitly addressed in the consent document itself. There are several relevant provisions in Utah law that apply here. Perhaps it was thought that there was no need to address it because there is a Utah statute on the issue of informed consent that provides that when the patient is incompetent, a relative (the statute lists the spouse) will be deemed to have the authority to act. Nevertheless, it would seem to me that this is an issue that one would want to discuss with a patient to draw out the patient's views and wishes. Although it may have been discussed, it was not reflected in what is called "the special consent form" (see appendix A), which the IRB approved as the satisfactory framework for the implant team's interaction with its first patient-subject.

Also, Utah law makes provision for what is called a durable power of attorney. Utah is one of forty-two states that have such statutes.[7] In examining the issue of the incompetent (but formerly

competent) patient, the President's Commission for the Study of
Ethical Problems in Medicine and Biomedical and Behavioral Research reached the conclusion that the durable power of attorney
statutes offer a very attractive means for dealing with medical uncertainty, especially in comparison with so-called living wills or other
forms of instruction-directives, as they are called, which provide
"this is what I want to have happen when this or that happens" but
which have a limited use because of a person's inability to anticipate
many possible situations in which life-or-death decisions must be
made. In contrast, the durable power of attorney statutes permit a
person to appoint someone to act on his or her behalf whose power
survives the point at which the appointer becomes incompetent. I
suspect that such an alternative would have offered some peace of
mind to the university implant team if it had sought legal advice and
desired to make clear in the eventuality that decisions had to be
made when Dr. Clark was incompetent that someone especially designated by him for this purpose would have had the specific authority, as provided in the statute, to step into his shoes and make the
full range of decisions about his treatment or its cessation.

Privacy

The final legal issue that I want to address is the question of privacy, specifically the control over publicity, most obviously as it
affected Dr. Clark and his family but also as it affected the professionals who were involved. Again, I must start with the available
documents, being an outsider to the process. Paragraph 15 of the special consent form discusses the sharing of information about Dr.
Clark with the world at large, and it states his consent thereto. The
form addresses the admittance of medical students and other medical observers in accordance with the ordinary practices of the university hospital; the use of videotaping through closed-circuit television; the taking of photographs, including motion pictures; the
preparation of drawings and similar graphic material; and the use of
these graphic materials for scientific purposes. It also mentions, as is
required by federal law, that the FDA will have access to the data
from this experiment. (What that really means is that the FDA insists
on access to the patient records.) "No public use," it goes on, "of
these materials will be made for purposes other than scientific presentation, and my rights to privacy and medical confidentiality will
be maintained, except by explicit permission from me or my authorized representative." That explicit permission is contained in a
separate statement, "Permission for Photographing, Filming, and/or
Interviewing Patient":

I authorize the University of Utah Hospital and/or a news agency to make a photograph or film of Dr. Barney B. Clark that may be used in a newspaper article, a television broadcast or a movie.

I consent to the use of my name, likeness or voice for such purposes, and I release the University of Utah officers, agents and employees, from all claim of liability with respect to the showing and use of such film or photograph.

Despite this bland and formal language, we are all aware of the folders full of newspaper and magazine clippings, to say nothing of the many videocassettes, in which Barney Clark was portrayed and discussed. Whether what actually happened would have been in a person's contemplation from the reference to "*a* newspaper article, *a* television broadcast or *a* movie" (italics mine), I leave to your own conclusions. It does seem to me that the language in the so-called special consent form and in the permission for photographing form is simply archaic. It bears no relationship to what happened here, in which the details of all aspects of Barney Clark's life, the lives of his wife and other people, even to his daily activities, were reported on national news. One could not turn on the television without knowing whether he was still having nosebleeds, whether he had exercised that day, or whether he recognized his wife when he emerged from an anesthetic.

Furthermore, the physicians themselves must also have felt that they were under intense public scrutiny, which is an unusual situation for physicians. This is very different from the practice strongly encouraged by Franz Ingelfinger and carried on by Arnold Relman, as editors of the *New England Journal of Medicine*: matters of medical investigation are to be carried on in private; after careful peer review they should first be reported in properly refereed professional journals (specifically, of course, in their journal!); and only thereafter should they be discussed in the general press.

I suppose that this issue of the traditions of medical privacy and of scientific investigation gets entwined here with some very special issues of the proprietary interests that are involved, both the proprietary interest of the physicians and also of the family, which we are now told finds itself engaged in a contract with *Reader's Digest* that, on a voluntary basis, limits the ability of members of the University of Utah team to have discussions with other people that will lead to published accounts in book form. Additionally, despite all the disclaimers, the Clark family apparently sees a limit to the amount of publicity covered in Dr. Clark's consent, since I was told by a member of the University administration that Mrs. Clark has now notified the public TV group that filmed the entire process that she does not want them to broadcast the sequence showing her husband's heart being removed because she finds that sensational, and that she objects, on the grounds of privacy, to its being shown. So, I don't think that one could say that through the kind of legal language that was used, those who planned the implant even began to address and resolve all of the issues of privacy and confidentiality.

In summary, what I find interesting here from a legal vantage point—treatment termination, surrogate decision-making, and privacy—all revolve in a very important way around the issues of the communication process among the participants, a matter frequently addressed by Jay Katz.[8] In this regard, I am reminded of Reinhold Niebuhr's famous aphorism that man's capacity for justice makes democracy possible and man's propensity for injustice makes democracy necessary, which was paraphrased by Princeton theologian Paul Ramsey in his Beecher Lectures: "Man's capacity to become joint adventurers in a common cause makes the consensual relation possible; man's propensity to overreach this joint adventure even in a good cause makes consent necessary."[9] If the law is to have any role here, I hope it is a role that is conducive to full disclosure and discussion—not talking *at* patients but talking *with* patients—and to an anticipation, with the aid of a good lawyer, of some of the issues that go beyond the issues of consent.

NOTES

1. Mrs. Karp sued her husband's surgeons for medical malpractice, but the judge directed a verdict for the defendants because the plaintiff failed to introduce expert evidence of defendants' negligence. See *Karp v. Cooley*, 349 F.Supp. 827 (S.D. Tex. 1972), *aff'd*, 493 F.2d 408 (5th Cir.), *cert. denied*, 419 U.S. 845 (1974).

2. Guido Calabresi and Philip Bobbitt, *Tragic Choices* (New York: W. W. Norton, 1978).

3. Jay Katz and Alexander M. Capron, *Catastrophic Diseases: Who Decides What?* (New York: Russell Sage Foundation, 1975).

4. See Gilbert S. Omenn's comments in this book.

5. President's Commission for the Study of Ethical Problems in Medicine and Biomedical and Behavioral Research, *Securing Access to Health Care* (Washington, D.C.: Government Printing Office, 1983).

6. A similar problem attends the question of "success." As our earlier discussion revealed, there was no definition of success, although the 1973 report of the Artificial Heart Assessment Panel states: "Since an objective of

the initial clinical trials would be evaluation of the duration and quality of the extended life, younger rather than older patients may be optimal subjects. Difficult decisions will have to be made about the implications of 'one-month,' 'one-year,' 'five-year,' and 'ten-year' anticipated survivals following implantation, especially where the alternative, without implantation, is certain death in the immediate future" (National Heart and Lung Institute, Artificial Heart Assessment Panel, *The Totally Implantable Artificial Heart: Economic, Ethical, Legal, Medical, Psychiatric, and Social Implications* [Washington, D.C.: U.S. Department of Health, Education and Welfare, 1973]). In other words, a decade ago that panel urged that policy and standards be spelled out in advance.

7. President's Commission for the Study of Ethical Problems in Medicine and Biomedical and Behavioral Research, *Deciding to Forego Life-sustaining Treatment* (Washington, D.C.: Government Printing Office, 1983), p. 137.

8. Jay Katz, *The Silent World of Doctor and Patient* (New York: Free Press, 1984).

9. Paul Ramsey, *The Patient as Person* (New Haven, Conn.: Yale University Press, 1970), pp. 5–6.

Summary of Discussion on Governmental, Sociological, and Legal Issues

WILLIAM A. CHECK

The afternoon session closed with questions and comments from the audience following the papers presented by Dr. Gilbert S. Omenn on governmental involvement in applying innovative medical technologies, by Dr. Renée C. Fox on sociological aspects of the heart implant program, and by Professor Alexander Morgan Capron on legal issues that may arise in such endeavors. In addition, the discussion drifted to a topic slated for presentation in the evening program: the involvement of the media, including privacy, press coverage, and university responses to the public's need to know.

GOVERNMENT REGULATION AND MEDICAL INNOVATION

The discussion that followed Dr. Omenn's presentation centered on the tension between regulation and innovation. Dr. William DeVries expressed the concern that overregulation may stifle the innovative process. He gave two examples encountered during development of the artificial heart. The Food and Drug Administration (FDA), which regulates medical devices such as the artificial heart, wanted the University of Utah team to demonstrate that the device would continue to work if a recipient rode in a plane. So one of the researchers put a calf with a heart implant into the back of a pickup truck and drove the truck and calf into the mountains to 8,000 feet, where the air pressure is equivalent to that maintained in a jet aircraft. The heart worked. In the other instance, Dr. DeVries referred to an informal survey he had done of articles in the *Journal of the American Society of Artificial Internal Organs*. In 1978 80 percent of all papers were from the United States, he found. But in 1982 Europe and Japan combined accounted for more published research than the United States.

Dr. Eric Cassell addressed a more fundamental question—the lack of understanding of what promotes creativity in society. Even more worrisome, we have no profession that even studies this process. In addition, Dr. Cassell highlighted the difference between individual achievement and social progress. Social progress does not necessarily come from an environment conducive of individual progress, he pointed out. Dr. Omenn pointed to a partial answer to this problem, a bill sponsored by Senator Orrin Hatch of Utah that would establish centers for health promotion in schools of public health.

Dr. Ray White of the University of Utah commented on the amount of research being done by commercial companies in the area of basic genetic research. He believed that this might be a significant force for innovation. Dr. Omenn agreed that privately funded research was desirable but said that the amount of money involved is "trivial." For example, the corporate grant to Massachusetts General Hospital is $50–$70 million over ten years. This will be only a trifling addition to the amount of money spent nationally by the National Institutes of Health on basic research over that period. In addition, Dr. Omenn pointed out, most of this corporate money is targeted toward products or processes expected to become feasible in the near term, different from the purpose of government grants awarded for basic research sometimes long before application becomes feasible.

The social attitude toward innovation itself changes with time, said Dr. David Blumenthal. In the mid-1960s people thought that there was much research just waiting to be converted to applications. More recently there has been pressure on costs, so innovation is now regarded more as a force tending to increase the costs of medical care. This leads to the "innovation-is-wheel-spin" view, Dr. Blumenthal said. Unfortunately, we really have no good data on what fosters or hinders innovation, so these views are merely fashions rather than facts.

MORMONISM AS A FACTOR IN THE ARTIFICIAL HEART PROGRAM

Of all of the excellent ideas presented by Dr. Fox, one proved to be most provocative and controversial. It was her contention that several unique features of the artificial heart experience with Dr. Clark were due to the unconscious influence of the Mormon culture prevalent in the region. Dr. Fox suggested that the Mormon world view may have shaped the familial spirit of the team, their relatively democratic interactions, the optimism at the medical center, some of the special features of its institutional review board (IRB), the extreme devotion of team members to Dr. Clark and his wife, the ardor of their commitment to pushing forward the frontiers of medical progress, and the simultaneously pedagogic and pastoral style of Dr. Chase Peterson with the press.

But several members of the implant team had strong reservations about this interpretation. Dr. Robert Jarvik thought the analysis was "very wrong and very damaging." Assuming that the program was guided by religious influences could raise the question of whether religion influenced the selection of the candidate. The personal features highlighted by Dr. Fox actually showed the basic humanness of the implant team, rather than their Mormonism, said Dr. Jarvik, who asserted that the University of Utah researchers were not predominantly Mormons. "The team member [referred to by Dr. Fox] who came to the hospital with his children to visit Dr. Clark on New Year's Eve was me," Dr. Jarvik said. "We popped open a bottle of champagne—not a predominantly Mormon tradition."

Both Dr. Fox and Dr. Jarvik were partly correct in Dr. Peterson's view. Religion was not considered in choosing the first implant patient. But Dr. Peterson thought that Dr. Fox accurately described Mormon cultural and theologic principles, which undoubtedly motivated or influenced Barney and Una Loy Clark and some of the heart team.

On the other hand, Peterson asked, Can Mormon culture be presumed to be able to influence non-Mormon or non-religious or atheistic team members? Is Mormon culture some sort of Chinese empire that absorbs and converts all who come to conquer it? More likely, he suggested, Mormon culture is uniquely American. Although it may be more vigorously expressed in the 1980s in the Mormonland than in Marin County, it is basically American, and what Dr. Fox picked up as Mormon features were in truth the peaks of Americanism that permeate Mormonism. Dr. Jarvik concurred. Love of family and a respect for education, for instance, are values that are not exclusively Mormon. They are held strongly in Mormonism, but they are also present throughout the American social fabric.

Dr. Fox then attempted to clear up what she saw as a misunderstanding of her analysis. As a sociologist, she said, she was not only, or even primarily, referring to Mormonism in terms of certain conventional forms of religious behaviors and attitudes, such as belonging to a particular church, participating in its religious services, abiding by its religious practices, subscribing to its doctrine, or respecting its clerical authorities. She was dealing with something broader, less literal, and less manifest than how many members of the heart team are or are not Mormon. What she was concerned with was Mormonism as a community, a distinctive culture, and a way of life, in which the University of Utah, its medical center, and heart team are embedded and by which they are influenced, as are most things in Salt Lake City.

One of the unique features of Mormonism is, indeed, how American it is, Dr. Fox agreed. It is in many ways the most American of religions. It is the typical and yet magnified degree to which Mormonism is so American that lies at the heart of the ways in which it is both "the same" and "different."

As an example of how pervasive and tenacious the influence of culture and cultural tradition can be, Dr. Fox described a phenomenon that she encountered in the People's Republic of China while she was doing medical sociological research there in 1981. At Tianjin's First Central Hospital, she was introduced to what that hospital called its "total quality control" (TQC) system. Upon her return to the United States, when she described some of the patterned characteristics of the shortcomings control classification scheme of TQC to sinologist colleagues, they were impressed by how many of its key features resembled those of the morality books and ledgers of merit and demerit that were kept by individuals and families in China's Ming Dynasty. In the Marxist-Leninist-Maoist TQC system, then, Confucian, Taoist, and Buddhist influences lived inadvertently on. Said Dr. Fox, "This gives us a kind of perspective on what culture is, how deeply below the surface it runs, how it is outside the purview of people in the immediate situation, and how powerfully enduring it is."

Alexander Capron suggested that people listen carefully to Dr. Fox's distinction. Religion is not the same as ethos or culture, he emphasized. Although most people who live in Salt Lake City probably aren't aware of it, he suggested that the feeling in this city is different from other cities. For instance, he noted, there isn't a "Family Night" every Friday night in Boston. Of course, all large cities have their own distinctive personalities, reflecting historical, ethical, and religious roots. One can think of San Francisco, New Orleans, and Montreal as examples.

Denise Grady enunciated one of the issues underlying the extensive discussion: "If Dr. Fox's analysis [of Mormon influence] is true," she said, "it might have implications for transferring this technology to other areas of the country."

LEGAL CONSIDERATIONS

Among the legal issues raised by Professor Capron, the one that provoked the most discussion was the thorny question of terminating treatment. Dr. Cassell raised the hypothetical situation of a patient who has not been told he is a candidate for the artificial heart, but whose heart fails on the operating table during bypass surgery, for example, and who then awakens with the implant already in place. Such a person would be told that he has the right to ask that the heart be turned off. This scenario sounds a bit unusual, but would there be any problem with stopping the heart if such a patient requests it and his physician believes he means it?

Dr. DeVries said he personally would have no problem with honoring such a request. We can all turn off our biological machines, he said, but it would be messier than with Dr. Clark. The only problem Dr. DeVries would have is being sure the patient truly wanted the device stopped.

Capron questioned Dr. Peterson about a statement that had been made to the press to the effect that acquiescence by the University of Utah in Dr. Clark's use of the key to turn off the heart would have placed the university in a very difficult position. Had Dr. Peterson actually said that? Had he since changed his mind? If he had changed his mind, Capron agreed with the new position.

Dr. DeVries said he had had a long discussion with Dr. Clark and his wife about how the machine would be turned off. Dr. Clark apparently had no problem in his mind with that arrangement. Dr. DeVries said he shared the view that technological suicide was not different from traditional suicide and was a personal prerogative. But from the university's point of view, the university would bear some sort of responsibility because of the problem in accurately determining the patient's intentions.

Dr. DeVries compared the situation with that of a very sick patient. The family of a sick patient might say it wanted the patient to die. But most people would consider it unwise for the doctor to have a handshake agreement with the family on this point, much less a legal contract. Months later the family could be overcome with guilt and blame the doctor. It might even find, using hindsight reasoning, evidence in the chart that the doctor agreed to the death inappropriately.

Capron then pointed out that medical research malpractice suits are much more unlikely than clinical malpractice suits. He also suggested that the Utah team had a chance to set criteria for an acceptable and believable expression of intent to die on the part of a patient. Once such criteria are set, he suggested, the researchers should consult with the university's ethicists and lawyers in order to affirm that stopping therapy is not suicide. The refusal of therapy—innovative or standard—is not suicide. There is a great distinction between a patient who is "suicidal" and one who is mentally competent but decides at some point that it is preferable to die.

Dr. Cassell agreed that the Utah team should take the opportunity to set standards in advance to determine a credible expression of a wish to have therapy stopped. The nice thing about preset standards is that the patient knows what will be recognized. It gives the patient comfort that his wishes will be respected. "Ethically, stopping therapy is no different from not starting," Dr. Cassell affirmed.

But University of Utah law professor Leslie Frances was not so sure. She asked, "Does cutting the air line or turning off the machine qualify as suicide or ceasing treatment?" She said it might be better to treat this situation as suicide, but a sympathetic suicide. Dr. Cassell replied, "What if the patient in this case asked you to turn off the machine, would this be suicide?" Dr. Peterson asked what would happen if newspapers had printed a picture of Barney Clark cutting his own air line. Leslie Francis agreed that suicide, rightly or wrongly, has very negative connotations in our society.

Dr. Jarvik noted the tendency for a hospital to take responsibility over patients. The doctors, for instance, decide when the patient can be discharged from the hospital. But what if the patient is at home, having severe problems, and says, "Do what you can here, but I don't want to go back into the hospital." There is a tendency for the heart team, as bound as it is to the patient, to want to maintain its grip even after the patient leaves, Jarvik noted.

Dr. Albert Jonsen thought that the chapter on the quality of death in the 1972 report on the artificial heart program should be rewritten in light of the foregoing comments. When clinical researchers embark on a procedure that has a high risk, they should consider the quality of death beforehand. Because the heart team all wanted Dr. Clark to live so badly, said Jonsen, they may not have confronted the quality of his death completely. As it turned out, Clark's death was not a failure.

PRIVACY AND THE PRESS

The question of how medical centers handle press coverage of events of wide public interest led to a discussion of press coverage itself. Talk so far had centered on the ethical responsibilities of the researchers, said Dr. Blumenthal, but what about the ethics of the press? How much does the public have a right to know, he asked? This question becomes especially important when the pervasive presence of the press during the ongoing medical experiment threatens to influence aspects of the experiment itself, such as the quality of life of the patient or patient selection. For example, anticipation of intensive press coverage might tend to discourage the researchers from picking a shy person for the implant, Dr. Blumenthal suggested. Dr. DeVries verified that one criterion for selection of the heart recipient was that he was prepared to handle the publicity.

Dr. Blumenthal wondered whether the foreknowledge of ubiquitous publicity might even disqualify a potential recipient whose family did not project well or were not solidly optimistic about the procedure. A wave of negative publicity during the first implant could prejudice long-term success of the whole program and technology. Dr. Blumenthal posed the question, "Where do you draw the line between the personal interest of the experimenters and the long-term value of society?"

Dr. Peterson acknowledged that these and other questions about press coverage received considerable thought from the University of Utah administration before the implant. But many of the policies just grew, he said, and were not planned in detail ahead of time. For the next procedure, Peterson believes that the university should decide on a more detailed course of action with regard to publicity.

The initial course was dictated by the belief that "the hospital was defenseless with respect to the press," Dr. Peterson said. The press couldn't be kept at bay. So university officials and the heart team decided to be as open as possible, trying to give "coherence" to the experience.

In addition, a secondary theme the university considered to be important was to provide some education about research that would have lasting value beyond the implant itself. This led to the university's providing the press with expert consultants, which the press accepted willingly.

One negative aspect of openness existed: it made the decision to terminate the human experiment potentially more difficult. For the next implant, that question will need to be thought through more carefully. Dr. Peterson described the University of Utah's approach to the release of public information about the implant as process logic. "This is a very western concept," he said, only half in jest. "We know we're taking the wagon somewhere, we just don't know where we're taking it."

PART THREE

Relations with the Media and the Institutional Review Board

After Barney Clark: Reflections of a Reporter on Unresolved Issues

LAWRENCE K. ALTMAN

The story that dominated news reports throughout the world 1 December 1982, and in the many days thereafter, came from the University of Utah Medical Center. It is a story that has brought us together for these days, and it is a story that is bound to unite us in other ways in the future.

But from the journalistic point of view, the story about Dr. Barney B. Clark's artificial heart implant operation did not begin in the closing hours of November 1982. It really began several years before when the University of Utah Medical Center public relations staff announced to medical and science reporters and news organizations the details of the university's progress in the artificial organs program, particularly emphasizing its aim of developing a functional artificial heart. The public relations staff did just what it should have done—orchestrated a news-organization march on Salt Lake City to cover the progress of the research that made Dr. Clark's operation possible.

My distinguished colleague, Harold M. Schmeck, Jr., made one of those trips here in 1981. It came about as follows: *New York Times* editors read a story on the wires stating that the University of Utah Institutional Review Board for Research with Human Subjects (IRB) was about to decide whether or not to allow the Utah heart team to proceed with an artificial heart implant. The editors decided it was an important development, and Harold came out here to write the story. Thereafter, Harold stayed in Salt Lake City to write another story for the Science Times section, this one on the artificial heart itself. Clearly, by publishing those two articles, the *New York Times* signaled how important it considered the potential of an artificial heart implant.

Another measure of the public interest in this developing technology: Harold was told that, after his original story appeared, representatives of all the major television networks called the University of Utah to complain that they had not been invited to the meeting of the IRB at which the decision was made. Harold replied that the University of Utah had nothing to worry about because if the television networks had been doing their jobs and had watched the wires they would have known enough to send someone out there in the first place.

So, as early as 1981, it was clear that the major news organizations were going to play the artificial heart implant as a major story. But those were not the only clear and unmistakable clues about the degree of the public's interest in the artificial heart. You had your own clues.

One was reflected in a story related by both Chase Peterson and Bill DeVries. Since they are present at this meeting, they can correct any errors in the version I am about to tell. My understanding was that while Bill was in the operating room one day, a call came from South America. The caller wanted to know if Bill would consider taking a certain patient as an artificial heart candidate. By the time Bill had lunch in the cafeteria, the cashier asked him if he was going to do the implant operation on that South American.

Word had spread so fast that it was unmistakable to Bill and Chase that the artificial heart implant operation could not be done secretly. Chase and Bill both told me that they had given fleeting thought to doing the operation secretly, Russian style. If it was successful, they would announce it after the event. If it failed, they would publish it in the *Journal of Negative Results* in another century or so. But the incident I related made it clear that secrecy was impossible. They said they settled on the NASA (National Aeronautics and Space Administration) approach, and we will come back to the NASA analogy later.

Given that background, it is hard to imagine how so many of you here at the University of Utah failed to anticipate the news media onslaught that came with Dr. Clark's hospitalization and subsequent surgery. Yet just about everyone I talked with here when I covered the Barney Clark story told me that they were flabbergasted at the media turnout as well as the amount of attention his story drew. Virtually all of us in the press corps were startled by the naïveté of that surprise.

After all, how is it that a medical school can invite the media, get the advance publicity it requested from virtually all major American news organizations, and then not expect them all to show up when the real event occurs? Journalists are human and are not known for enjoying coitus interruptus. So the attitude of surprise lies some-where between naïveté and incompetence.

Well, what happened after we all came here? We found that you were not well prepared, at least from the news media perspective. You earned mixed grades for your efforts. Part of the problem may have been due to the circumstances of Dr. Clark's case—that he stayed in the hospital for 112 days, much longer than anyone ex-pected. Even so, much of what has transpired since Dr. Clark's ad-mission to the University of Utah Medical Center—and it is just shy of a year now—confirms that impression.

I was asked to speak here tonight on the topic "After Barney Clark: Unresolved Issues and Reflections of a Reporter Who Covered the Artificial Heart Implant Story." I think the simplest way of doing that will be to raise a number of questions by topics. I am not going to answer the questions because my prime purpose will be in pro-voking all of us to think about them. Please take them in that spirit. There are nine topics, as follows: news conferences; scientific re-ports; public relations; the University of Utah IRB; commercialism; the NASA analogy; history of the Utah artificial heart models; follow-up; and the second case.

NEWS CONFERENCES

The highest marks go to Chase Peterson for his extraordinary handling of the news conferences. What made them work was Chase's imagination, his ability to speak so articulately, as well as his instant command of vivid analogies. Some of his analogies may not have been precise; never mind that he stumbled occasionally. When he did, the manufacturers of chicken soup loved him! Still, his batting average would have led any major league. And it is doubt-ful that anyone else could have done any better, if as well, as did Chase. From the public relations point of view, he was the Univer-sity of Utah's star.

Moreover, you deserve high marks for carrying out at least one aspect of the NASA analogy. You announced the major medical devel-opments in Dr. Clark's case. When crises occurred, you let us know. You said that in so many hours we will send Dr. Clark back to the operating room. And then you told us what happened. Hurrah!

Clearly, you faced a few problems and you handled them well. If you did not know how diversified a field journalism is, you found out almost instantly in the cafeteria news room. No one could deny that we were a motley crew. There were reporters whose greatest concern seemed to be, shall we say, the color of Dr. Clark's pajamas. These reporters also wanted to know their size! And what's more, even if you had given a straightforward, simple answer—blue, extra large, and from Brooks Brothers—you knew that there would be one reporter popping up to demand a shorter, simpler answer! Then, there were some of us who wanted the laboratory values and other clinical facts to make our reports more scientific. We wanted the value of the hematocrit, creatinine, and other tests, not the size of the pajamas!

Well, you did not gather here just for praise; otherwise, you would not have originally scheduled this as a closed meeting. So let us concentrate on the problems—the major unresolved questions of Dr. Clark's case.

SCIENTIFIC REPORTS

As we approach the first anniversary of Dr. Clark's artificial heart implantation, I am unaware of any scientific report that has appeared in any medical journal. I am astonished.

Dr. Christiaan Barnard's first heart transplant operation in 1967 certainly received as much publicity as Dr. William DeVries' first case. Yet it took less than one month for Dr. Barnard's report to appear in a peer-reviewed journal, the *South African Medical Journal*. The operation was performed on 3 December 1967, and the report of the first case appeared in the 30 December issue of the *South African Medical Journal*. The same issue carried a report of the autopsy as well as another report on the legal requirements of the acquisition of human tissue for transplantation purposes in South Africa.

Given the speed with which the first heart transplant was reported to the scientific profession, we must ask why there have not been any published scientific reports of the first artificial heart case beyond the ones presented orally at a few specialty meetings in Atlanta and Toronto and perhaps a few other places.

When I spoke with Dr. DeVries last April he told me that the team was just about to send off a report to the *New England Journal of Medicine*. I presume the report was sent. The question is, Why hasn't it appeared yet in that journal or any other?

I don't know the answer, but in analyzing the problem it is obvious that one possibility is that, countrary to what I was told, the Utah paper was never submitted to the *New England Journal of*

Medicine or any other scientific publication. If that is the case, why the change of mind? Why hasn't the scientific community been informed?

Another possibility is that the reports have just been sent off to a journal. If so, it raises the key question, Why the delay? Or, if not, why haven't they been submitted for publication?

Still another possibility is that the paper was rejected. If so, why was it rejected? Were the objections for reasons of scientific merit? Or was the rejection on the basis of the so-called Ingelfinger-Relman rule?[1]

When I tried to learn the answer to this question last summer through the University of Utah Medical Center's news office, I was told it was none of the press's business. I disagree. It is the business of the press to report the developments and steps, controversial or not, in the process of reporting such a historic case.

The problems involved in doing a historic case are as important as the collecting of scientific data, and yet these factors are seldom included in the scientific reports of discoveries and historic medical events. Scientific papers are usually written long after the laboratory experiments are finished or the case reports are prepared, long after diagnostic and treatment procedures are completed. And the scientific reports do not reflect the dead ends, blind alleys, and numerous wrong turns that doctors almost always take in such events. Scientific papers are usually written in a form that tries to make it clear that the authors knew exactly how they were proceeding from the very beginning. In short, there is an element of fiction in the medical literature. There's less chance of that here because the NASA approach was adopted. Still, reporters did not have the opportunity to question Dr. Clark directly.

I submit also that this practice of literary license does the scientific and medical communities a great disservice because we delude ourselves into believing that things happen that way and the public, told that discoveries are more clear-cut than they really are, comes to expect that research is a simpler process than it really is. Accordingly, doctors in succeeding generations have great difficulty in understanding how the tests, therapies, knowledge, and other like tools of trade that they have inherited got to be that way.

We also wanted to hear a lot more about the specifics of the science involved in Dr. Clark's case, not just the general statements indicating that the researchers have learned a lot scientifically. Specifically, what was learned? Most of us are still confused on this point.

If the journal papers were rejected on scientific grounds, then it seems there may be reason to question the validity of the experiment. But, if the journals rejected the paper because of the wide publicity given before scientific publication in the *New England Journal of Medicine* or some other publication with a similar rule, then I would like to hear from the ethicists and sociologists here about the impact of this policy regarding prior publicity as it applies in this case.

Whether or not the papers were rejected by the *New England Journal of Medicine*, it was clear that the impact of the Relman rule was felt in the news conferences. Members of the Utah heart team told me it was one of their concerns. Given that fact, let me raise some more questions for the ethicists, sociologists, and others here. What are the ethics of the restrictions imposed by medical journals on a research project of this type? And what effect does that have on the potential health care of Americans?

The most frequent comment I hear from cardiologists and medical leaders with whom I have discussed Dr. Clark's case is that they feel limited in what they have been able to learn about the case. Stated more bluntly, the cardiologists say that they do not have enough scientific information to discuss it in an intelligent way.

We have, then, a baffling situation. Doctors complain that they want their information first in medical journals. So apparently in compliance with that policy, the Utah heart team limited what it said about the science of the artificial heart case at the news conferences. But that leaves everyone in a peculiar, Catch-22 situation. The medical profession complains it cannot discuss the case intelligently because there hasn't been enough scientific data. And one possible explanation why there hasn't been enough data is that the medical journal has rejected the paper because there was too much publicity. And if the answer is because the papers have only just been sent off or have not yet been submitted, then we must ask, Is it a delaying tactic for commercial reasons—to somehow benefit Kolff Medical? If so, what are the ethics involved here in terms of a scientific project funded by taxpayer monies but being controlled by a private corporation?

PUBLIC RELATIONS

It is because the taxpayers paid for the development of the artificial heart and the University of Utah is a public institution that public relations is so important in telling Dr. Clark's story as well as other aspects of the artificial heart program. Let me remind you that in this post–World War II era, the taxpayer, the public, has become the chief benefactor of medicine. Medicine is now a public institution because it is the taxpayer who is paying for the bulk of the costs of patient care, medical research, and medical education. Members of the medical profession have become public servants. And they are accountable to the public in the same way that other public servants are.

If you have come to think of the artificial heart as a private venture because Kolff Medical is controlling it, I think you are overlooking some basic facts. The federal Food and Drug Administration must approve what you are doing. The taxpayers through the National Institutes of Health are paying for most of the related current and future research at the University of Utah. Moreover, if the artificial heart proves successful in further experiments, the choice of whether or not to pay for the implants as a standard medical procedure will be up to the American public, not you. That is because the American taxpayer funds Medicare and similar health insurance programs.

Let me remind you that what the public understands about Dr. Clark's case and the artificial heart is through what you tell the media and the public. You are the only ones who knew what actually happened because you were there. But, as John Dwan has said, you chose to control the release of that information to the public. And because of that, you are subject to the leaks that inevitably occur in such situations. When there are leaks, you are subject to the distortions that can go with them. I am not saying that such distortions have occurred. I am simply pointing out the problem to you.

The only thing that news reporters can report is what we are told and what we learn about what we have been told. We are outsiders looking in, always questioning, because we did not have the primary experience. So, we have to ask an unpleasant but fundamental question: Were the flaws and attitudes expressed by the problems in presenting Dr. Clark's case to the public a tip-off about the quality of administration and research involved in the artificial heart research?

Don't forget that you told us in early news conferences that Barney Clark was the ideal candidate for the artificial heart. A special independent university committee (the IRB) gave the necessary unanimous approval for Dr. Clark. Now the head of the Utah IRB considers Dr. Clark not to have been the ideal candidate. Yet we have not had an adequate explanation from the IRB about why he was not the ideal candidate.

THE INSTITUTIONAL REVIEW BOARD

One of the most important but least discussed aspects of the Barney Clark case is the role of the IRB. We all know that, according to a federal mandate, IRBS exist at each medical center where research is supported by the federal government. There are at least 550 IRBS, perhaps even 1,000, in the United States, and there seem to be few formal rules that govern them all. For the most part, IRBS operate in similar ways although there are considerable local variations, and the University of Utah's IRB seems to have some unusual features.

Since IRBS are federally mandated and the IRB here has considerable clout over the artificial heart experiment, the public has a right to ask some basic questions about this group. First, one IRB member, Dr. Ross Woolley, has said that he spent up to four hours with Dr. Clark each of the 112 days after the implant operation. Dr. Woolley said he attended rounds, read the chart, and participated in discussions. He also, I am told, gave a blessing when Dr. Clark died.

When I mentioned all of this to several members of other IRBS in this country, they expressed astonishment. In a small sample, I could find no one who knew of a similar situation. IRB members are not known to continually witness experiments, although some do conduct spot checks. Dr. Woolley's presence struck some members of IRBS elsewhere as a vigilante or policing role. At least it could be perceived as such. Accordingly, we reporters have some unanswered questions:

1. How much of a threat to the Utah heart team did the constant presence of a member of the IRB represent? Is a policing role a proper one for IRB members? On the other hand, was it a good thing? Should it be repeated?

2. Who was, and is, running the artificial heart experiment at the University of Utah? The heart team or the IRB?

3. If there is so much controversy now about the selection of Dr. Clark and so much delay in getting basic facts to the IRB for its consideration of a second patient, why has it taken so long, given the fact that Dr. Woolley was there all the time?

4. A videotaped interview with Dr. Clark was released publicly and shown widely on national television. The interview was billed as one between Dr. DeVries and Dr. Clark. But few know that a third person was involved in that interview. Several of the questions were asked by Dr. Woolley, not Dr. DeVries, yet this was never publicly disclosed. Why?

From the public's perspective, that interview was one of the most striking and controversial aspects of Dr. Clark's case. It was the only time the public saw him with his artificial heart, and to most he came off looking like a zombie. Dr. Clark looked like he was staring off into space, unable to look at Dr. DeVries, his interviewer.

When I reviewed the videotapes with John Dwan, he told me, in answer to my question, that Dr. Clark was looking directly at Dr. Woolley. Dr. Woolley? No one said he was interviewing Dr. Clark. Since IRBs were set up to help resolve ethical problems, we must ask what is the ethics of that? Was it proper not to identify Dr. Woolley? Was his role as an interviewer a proper one for an IRB member?

5. Was it fair to Dr. Clark that his viewers did not know that he was not staring into space as a zombie but instead was looking at Dr. Woolley? What are the ethics of that situation?

6. John Dwan and others told me that the videotape was made at the end of the day, a time when Dr. Clark was usually at his weakest. Moreover, it was made on a day when he had had an unusually hectic schedule. Why was there no better planning for this, his only public exposure after he got the artificial heart? Was that filming fair to future applicants for the artificial heart? How well did this lone, edited videotape serve the memory of Dr. Clark?

7. What is the proper role of the IRB in the artificial heart experiment? Dr. Woolley told two other journalists and me that the IRB's role was to protect the institution. He has used the term "institutional integrity" in talking to others. Now that seems odd since the original idea was for IRBs to protect the research volunteer and patient from institutional overreaching. Again, in my spot check with other IRB members I find no support for the position. Should there be? I think we need some discussion of this point at this meeting.

I learned only today that Dr. DeVries invited Dr. Woolley to monitor the patient and that Dr. Woolley no longer votes on the artificial heart on the IRB. But I do not know when this change occurred and why we weren't told about it.

To the best of my knowledge, the IRB has held only one news conference during the entire artificial heart program. And that one was held in late September and was dubbed a "damage control" session because it was held a week or so after leaked statements from members of the IRB were televised locally and nationally.

It seems to me that the university created its own problems by not having IRB members discuss the progress of its deliberations publicly. If the deliberations were taking an extraordinarily long time, then the IRB should have told the public that that was the case and should have explained why.

Given the university's silence, no wonder people were surprised when they heard about the minority views expressed on television, even though they had been written about several months earlier. The university invited that type of leak.

In the recent IRB press conference, Dr. John Bosso (the chairman) maintained that the artificial heart represents a big advance in medical care and if proven successful could be of benefit to hundreds of thousands of patients in this country alone. For that reason, he said, the onus is on the University of Utah investigators and the IRB to move slowly and cautiously, with adequate documentation.

Few would argue with that approach. But I think many would have difficulty without further explanation of Dr. Bosso's statement that seven months after Dr. Clark's death the IRB still does not have sufficient information from Dr. DeVries to evaluate a new protocol. More important, it seems to me, is his statement that the IRB still does not know what information it needs to make such a decision.

Why doesn't the IRB have the information it needs? Why doesn't it know what information to seek? After all, a subcommittee was appointed to review all the procedures. Dr. Woolley, by his admission, spent every day with Dr. Clark. What did he do all that time? Why is the IRB in the dark about its needs?

Dr. Bosso says that many hours have been spent with the issue and that he will readily admit that it appears, from the outside, that the IRB is dragging its feet and not really doing anything but that the public will have to trust him and the IRB. Dr. Bosso also said that the IRB had been ineffectual in conveying its needs to Dr. DeVries. Dr. Bosso said: "If there has been a logjam in moving this ahead, it certainly has been the IRB for the most part, but I would certainly not apologize for that."

Well, let's think about that. If the artificial heart is as important as Dr. Bosso says it is, then I think the American public has a right to know exactly what has been going on in those deliberations and why they have taken so long.

Yes, IRBs are designed to protect volunteers from overzealous researchers. But there are critical questions here: Who protects volunteers and patients in need? Who protects the public from the procrastinations of an ineffective IRB? We need some discussion of those questions. Remember, all the deliberations of the IRB have been in secret. And when the media learn only a few facts, the IRB threatens to prosecute.

When I was covering Dr. Clark's case, I was told that the IRB met in closed sessions to discuss the artificial heart. When I asked if records were kept of those discussions and meetings, I was told that they were not. The leaked documents make it clear that I was not given the correct information. Why was the university not honest in answering the question? Why did the university create a needless credibility gap?

So we have to ask still some fundamental questions: Who is judging the quality of the IRB's review? To whom is the IRB accountable? How will historians and public officials be able to look back and judge the way the University of Utah handled the artificial heart research? Maybe the IRB wants no one to be able to judge its work. But I raise the question of the ethics of that attitude. Moreover, is that a proper way to conduct research?

Future generations need to know how and why research advances and fails. The documents involved in the IRB deliberations will be crucial not only to future heart research but also to research of all types. Recall that I said that much of what makes its way into the medical literature has a fictional element to it. Will that be the case here?

COMMERCIALISM

According to the informed consent form that Dr. Clark signed twice, he was responsible for the costs of his hospitalization. Apparently, no one expected him to stay in the hospital for as long as he did and for the care to have cost as much as it did—$250,000 according to the last accounting. We were led to believe by the grapevine that Dr. Clark made some poor investments. So, when the university announced that it was not going to hold Dr. Clark and his family responsible for the costs of his care, at first glance it seems to have been a very charitable move. But, we also learned that the Clark family signed a contract with *Reader's Digest* for an exclusive story about his ordeal. The amount of money has not been disclosed, to my knowledge.

Well, from the outside looking in, something is missing in the logic here. If the family was excused for paying the bill, then why did the family need the financial benefits of an exclusive arrangement? Why was checkbook journalism needed? What kind of a precedent has the University of Utah set for medical research?

But knowing that such an exclusive arrangement exists, we who are on the outside and who have no direct knowledge of the terms of the contract, again must ask some hard questions:

1. Is there a secret clause in the *Reader's Digest* contract that calls for a delay in publication of scientific papers or in choosing a second case? Have the scientific reports been held up for that reason?

2. Concerning the videotape of Dr. Clark's operation, is the *Reader's Digest* contract the reason why the Clark family has refused to allow it to be shown on a documentary television program? Why do we have a problem now? Why wasn't the issue clarified before the operation?

Why was the videotape made? What discussions were held about doing it? Who participated? Where are the minutes of those discussions? I heard that it cost $150,000 to make the videotape. Who paid that bill? Who controls the videotape? To whom has it already been shown? I have heard that Dr. Lyle Joyce showed it to a high school class. Is that true? Moreover, where is the line drawn between those who see it for educational purposes at the University of Utah and the public? Would all cardiac surgeons who wanted to see it be allowed to see it? If so, what about all thoracic surgeons? All general surgeons? All cardiologists? All physicians? Remember, there is good reason to show it to them because any among them could be potential referring physicians.

Kolff Medical has sought venture capital to finance its future activities. Members of other medical school faculties have either formed or joined genetic engineering companies just as several University of Utah faculty members have done with Kolff Medical. Some of these ventures represent radical changes from the usual academic activities. This leads to further questions:

1. Have the scientific reports been held up because of Kolff Medical's financial dealings?

2. To what extent is there a conflict of interest when members of the heart team hold shares in Kolff Medical?

3. What are the plans for Kolff Medical to work with the Hospital Corporation of America, Temple University, Baylor University, and other groups? If the University of Utah IRB rejects a protocol for a second artificial heart, will the team move elsewhere?

For those who think I am too harsh, recall that we reporters found it nearly impossible to ascertain the name of the valve that broke in Dr. Clark's artificial heart. At the time, we were told that the manufacturer would not be revealed because Dr. Jarvik and Dr. Kolff had had such good dealings with them and also because people who had those valves in their hearts would worry too much. I submit that that is not a valid reason for not discussing the valve problem more openly. When I tried to interview Dr. Kolff on the subject he told me I should know better than to ask questions I knew he would not answer. He no longer gives interviews because of the *Reader's Digest* contract.

What is the financial arrangement between Kolff Medical and the valve's manufacturer? Why shouldn't that be public knowledge?

The broken valve raises another question: A broken valve was clearly a possibility in the planning of the first artificial heart operation. Why wasn't the heart team more open in providing the data about the number of broken valves in the animal experiments before Dr. Clark received his heart? Did the team tell Dr. Clark how many valves broke? Did the IRB know? If not, why not? How can we determine that fact? What are the ethics of not disclosing that information to the patient and to the public?

THE NASA ANALOGY

Drs. Peterson and DeVries used the NASA analogy several times, so let's think about it. The analogy, it seems to me, has only limited application to the artificial heart case. But they used it in much broader terms. It does apply to the fact that the university announced the operation in advance and reported the complications as they occurred. But it does not apply in the sense that in the space program the public could listen to the air-to-ground communications between the astronauts and the space officials at the very same time that the space officials were learning what was going on. The public was not tuned into the operating room when Dr. Clark's heart was being removed. Nor should the public have been there at that time unless the recipient specifically requested it. However, the videotape was made. And there is a case for showing excerpts of it publicly. If the NASA analogy holds, then it follows that the public should see it, regardless of Mrs. Clark's views.

Further, NASA presented the scientific findings as they occurred in press conferences and then published scientific papers. You did not, at least to the same extent, present the scientific data at news conferences. And we have yet to see the scientific papers.

HISTORY OF THE UTAH ARTIFICIAL HEART MODELS

Not until 5:30 last night did I learn the answer to a question I asked last winter, and then the answer came by accident. Several of us had wondered how the Jarvik-7 model number had been chosen. We wondered how this model differed from the Jarvik-1 or Jarvik-4 or other like models. I could get no answer to my question, and I looked for a background paper in the press kit. There was none on the point. So I, and I believe many others, got the impression that it was a number selected much like Boeing and other airline companies choose to call planes a 707 or 747 or Korean Air Lines chooses flight 007.

The point was reinforced by your latest news release that described the implantation of the Utah 100. The news release gave no explanation of why the model number was chosen, and the public relations staff, when asked, did not know the answer. What about the missing models from Jarvik-7 to Utah 100?

Then on the tour yesterday, Dr. Don Olsen mentioned that the Utah 100 has a stroke volume of 100 cc of blood and the Utah 85, 85 cc. That was a partial explanation but the Jarvik-7 also has a stroke volume of 100 cc. And then we were shown the museum with all the models back to Dr. Kolff's first in the 1950s. All it would have taken to answer our question was a photograph of that exhibit. The photograph and a chronological history could have been handed out to the news corps.

It is a small point in one way but not in another. Had you done it, we could have written stories about the many predecessors of the Jarvik-7, why it took so long to get there, an insight into the blind alleys, an education of the benefactor, the public, of what research is really like. But with all the advance warning, you still did not prepare yourselves. The university had a chance to do a little education—after all that is its basic purpose—but it didn't. Last night after our meeting one university official, in discussing some of these issues, told me I should not have expected such preparation from the university or the public relations office. I was extremely disappointed to learn his views.

There's another possibly important point here. During the course of the first implant, members of the news media began hearing from Dr. Clifford S. Kwan-Gett and his dispute over credit for priority in developing the artificial heart. Then, suddenly, the university began calling the Jarvik-7 the Utah heart. We have not had a full airing of the priority dispute. Perhaps some of this would have been avoided if the university had issued a background paper on the history of the development of the models.

FOLLOW-UP

The essence of good clinical medicine and research is the quality of the follow-up. The same holds true in journalism.

University of Utah officials repeatedly said that the press would be notified of significant developments in the course of the artificial heart story. In the specific case of Dr. Clark, the media were asked to stay away from the family in return for the guarantee of being told what was going on. When I left here last April after Dr. Clark's death, I was told that this policy would hold for future developments as well.

Well, significant events have transpired without, to the best of my knowledge, any news releases. Dr. Jarvik has left the university to become president of Kolff Medical. The university now owns quite a few shares of Kolff Medical, and agreements have been made with other hospital chains and universities. Yet we haven't been told much about them.

There are dangers to releasing partial information and controlling the information. We had heard nothing from the IRB until its only news conference. We did not know that Dr. Woolley had joined the heart team or that he was invited to be on the ward by Dr. DeVries. And yet this information is pertinent to the telling of the ongoing story.

Dr. Woolley said he saw the artificial heart as the focus of serious discussions of ethics, how society would provide health care to people, and so forth, in the next few years. How, I ask, can that be the case when we know very little—really nothing—of the IRB's activities and deliberations?

THE SECOND CASE

I have heard it said several times that the media's and public's fascination with the artificial heart will rapidly fade with the second case and that the media attention will be much less. Maybe this will be true, but I'm not so sure. There might be even more interest than in Dr. Clark's case.

The way you have controlled the release of the scientific information and the IRB reports, you have created much more controversy than ever existed. The story is much more interesting now. The public now has many more questions about the program than it did before. Moreover, if the second patient goes home, then the interest will be even greater than it was in Dr. Clark's case.

Recent developments at the University of Utah raise much more important questions. There have been several administrative changes made since Dr. Clark's death. Moreover, there has been a key turnover in the surgical team: Dr. Lyle Joyce, the second in command, has left the University of Utah. How can you proceed the next time so shortly after the number two surgeon has gone? Who will be second in the second operation? Kolff Medical's prospectus makes the point very clear: a highly trained surgical team is required to implant an artificial heart. Will that person be adequately trained and have enough experience if the second case is done in the next few weeks?

Even if Dr. Joyce returns for the second operation, as has been suggested, then for how long can he stay in Salt Lake City during the postoperative period? For 112 days? If the convalescence took as long as Dr. Clark's and Dr. Joyce stayed only part of the period, would that be good care? Can Dr. Joyce suddenly abandon his patients in Minneapolis to come to Salt Lake City to help the artificial heart team?

If someone other than Dr. Joyce is the second, and the second implant fails, might the fact that a new number two surgeon was involved in the operation be potential grounds for a malpractice suit? Should it be? We ought to have some discussion of these issues.

It is impossible for one individual to cover all of the unresolved issues. I am sure other members of the press could add a number of other points for discussion.

I have intended these remarks to be provocative and to fulfill my assigned task of raising questions for later discussion at the conference. Since I believe that journalism is a two-way street, I do not consider myself immune from attack. So I would be willing to tackle some of the questions you may have, if you have any.

Thank you.

NOTE

1. The Ingelfinger-Relman rule is a policy of the *New England Journal of Medicine* that was formulated by former editor Franz Ingelfinger and extended by the present editor Arnold Relman. It holds that proffered papers may not be accepted for publication if the details have been reported previously in the news media.

A Spontaneous Reply to Dr. Lawrence Altman

CHASE N. PETERSON

I had not planned to respond to Dr. Lawrence Altman's presentation, but it is clear that a response is required. Larry has raised some very searching questions about critical issues in the heart program, and it is important that we try to answer them. He has raised both speculative ideas and specific issues that we need to address. There is no progress if we don't learn from criticism, and his questions deserve answers.

I suppose, Larry, that if we had asked you to act as a paid consultant to the heart team, you would have raised these same probing questions. Of course, it would have been easier to deal with them inside a university board room, but since we are in a forum here for discussion and since our exchange will be published, perhaps the challenge has, in a sense, been sharpened for us.

I have about one hundred answers here on this small piece of paper. You have the questions. The answer to number 37 is no! Seriously, we need to address our underestimate of media interest. We weren't entirely surprised nor were we entirely unprepared. You rightfully pointed out that we welcomed the media with briefings on the animal experimental program more than a year earlier. John Dwan, Anne Brillinger, and Pam Fogel, from our public affairs office, were convinced that there would be intense interest on the part of the media, and they made plans to make your stay as comfortable as possible. We put in dozens of phones, set aside space in the cafeteria, and planned the food service. However, we were surprised by the large number of media representatives who came from all over the world and stayed. We expected they would leave several days after the operation, file their stories, and edit their film. Instead, they stayed, many of them, throughout the long 112 days until Dr. Clark's death. So you are both right and wrong. We anticipated and we prepared, but it wasn't enough.

NEWS CONFERENCES

We decided in advance that it would be both inappropriate and impossible to conduct the heart experiment in secret, so we opened ourselves to criticism and scrutiny throughout. Of course we were concerned about the Clark family's privacy, but we and they believed that intrusive questions from the press were proper and were to be expected. I am not aware of any scientific experiment in which so much information was divulged as the experiment unfolded. We didn't cover the story in the same detail that would be expected in a scientific article, but our disclosures were direct and accurate and honest and we stand on the record. We think there is educational value in reporting a dramatic human experiment in lay language. After all, education is the raison d'être of a university. We think we were successful in advancing the understanding of medical experiments, and as you pointed out, contemporary disclosures run a much smaller risk of being sanitized than scientific articles written for professional journals. In these papers you read the clean results with data and graphs and carefully selected illustrations, but the researcher doesn't write about all of the mistakes made along the way. Is it not true that we shared our mistakes and our ignorance with you? Those hourly reports, when Barney Clark had subcutaneous emphysema, are an example. We didn't know the cause at first and we said so. I remember talking to Bill DeVries and Lyle Joyce and Rob Jarvik about four possible explanations for the crepitation. Then Bill and Lyle went to the operating room to find out what was causing it while I went to the briefing room to outline the four possibilities and bring reporters up to date on our thinking at this stage. Bill told me later that, as he was coming out of the operating room with Dr. Clark on the gurney, he looked up at the television set with interest to find out what I was telling them in the newsroom. In his jocular way he said, "I was pleased to learn what it was that I had been doing." As a matter of fact, Bill checked and ruled out the first three possible causes that I had written on the blackboard, and he found the fourth—ruptured alveolar blebs—which he promptly repaired. That direct approach lets people know that doctors are not Olympian gods who get insights by inspiration; they have to search and rule out various options and alternatives. That was the way we viewed our role in the news conferences.

SCIENTIFIC REPORTS

I am happy to report that the *New England Journal of Medicine* has a complete article, which Dr. Arnold Relman tells me has been accepted. I spoke to him just a week and a half ago. In fact, he wanted to join us in our conference here but couldn't clear his calendar. He even hoped he could have it in print before this conference, but obviously hasn't been able to do so.[1] Bill DeVries has a case study in press in the *Journal of Thoracic and Cardiovascular Surgery*, and it will be coming out shortly.[2]

As an aside, I have never forgiven Larry for his confusion between my literary metaphors and his sense of science with respect to chicken soup. We were discussing what could cause seizures in a person who was in acute renal failure in the diuretic phase. I am an old nephrologist, and I know that in diuresis it is very common to have multiple metabolic imbalances. Under these circumstances the body requires a variety of things to choose from and ultimately will retain what it needs—calcium, magnesium, or something else— to bring itself back into balance. So, as the metaphor went—evidently a metaphor too sophisticated for the *New York Times*—I told the press that we were going to feed him chicken soup to correct his metabolic imbalance. If you had ever read Maimonides, Dr. Altman, you would know that "the soup of the fat chicken" is curative. In any case, chicken soup was the metaphor to suggest that what we were going to give him was a range of nutrients from which his body could choose.

By the way, Hal Wolf, the university's dean of pharmacy, was in Los Angeles the next week at a convention, and he had a tag on his lapel that read "The University of Utah." The word was circulating that chicken soup had some relationship to Barney Clark's seizures. The waiter serving Hal kept going back and forth, looking at his name tag, and finally he got the nerve to ask, "Excuse me sir, but my boy has epilepsy. What brand of chicken soup do you use at the University of Utah?" Really, Larry, there was no suggestion that fatty chicken soup was being given intravenously to Barney Clark.

PUBLIC RELATIONS

It seems to me that we are being blamed for some of the leaks that occurred that led to erroneous rumors, but at the same time we are not being given proper credit for having told as much as we did. If we had clammed up entirely we would have been prone to many more leaks. That there were so few leaks only documents my argument that openness is better than secrecy.

As you know, one of the leaks occurred just a few weeks ago when it was reported that the University of Utah Institutional Review Board (IRB) had serious questions about Barney's suitability as a heart implant candidate because of his chronic obstructive pulmonary disease. The IRB had not been fully informed that Barney's pulmonary problems were determined to be mild prior to surgery. Dr. Terence Block in Seattle and Dr. Jeffrey Anderson here both agreed with that opinion. He had never required bronchodilators. Now half of the people in this room have, at some time, used bronchial dilators for asthma, wheezing, or bronchitis. But he never took them and he never required oxygen. The cardiac catheterization studies revealed relatively greater failure of the left ventricle than of the right ventricle. It is the right ventricle that fails when there is lung disease. Furthermore, the artificial heart is uniquely qualified to compensate for right ventricle failure because it can pump through a stenotic pulmonary artery or a scarred lung, whereas a normal heart or a transplanted heart cannot. There was no way to distinguish how much of his pulmonary disease was secondary to heart failure and how much was primary. Of course it is impossible to state that Barney Clark was the "perfect" case because he did have some lung disease. We acknowledged during Barney Clark's postoperative life that we were disappointed to find the extent of his pulmonary disease at the time of surgery. But I would argue that if he presented himself as a candidate again with the studies and observations we had from his admitting physicians, he would be chosen again because of the evidence that he had only mild chronic obstructive pulmonary disease.

In summary, I believe that our public relations were good, but of course they could have been better and we intend to try to improve.

THE INSTITUTIONAL REVIEW BOARD

A major issue here is that whenever you set up an independent institution there is the danger that it will become autonomous to the point of being irresponsible. As an example, the Utah Supreme Court has had a case pending for two years concerning the taxability of public hospitals. It is a terribly important issue that needs to be resolved. What pressures can be put upon the court? None. What pressures should be put to bear? None, I would argue, except perhaps a little bit of public pressure. There really is no way that one can, or should, interfere with court proceedings.

Now, how do IRBs operate? They work independently. What kinds of pressure should be put on them? None. They are set up by federal guidelines; they are set up within the university; and once they are established, there is no way that the university could or should put pressure on their decisions. So when the question is asked, Why don't we know what the IRB is doing? the answer is because we don't want to know what the IRB is doing, any more than we want to know what the Supreme Court is doing with respect to some case that is before it. That is the price you pay for autonomy. Because the IRB is designed to protect the interests of patients who are research subjects, we think it is very important that autonomy of the IRB is the primary concern, the IRB's sense of responsibility to the university is secondary, and loyalty is a nonissue.

I think the fact that the University of Utah IRB chose to have closed meetings instead of open ones is a matter of discretion on its part. It does not qualify as an infringement of academic freedom, as you seem to suggest, Larry. Academic freedom is the freedom to think and to write and to teach, and it has nothing to do with the concepts of privacy and confidentiality. It was the IRB's business to decide whether or not to hold open meetings and whether or not to take minutes of its meetings. I don't know why you were told that members were not taking minutes, if they were. The University of Utah protects the rights of its faculty—the freedom to think, write, teach, or talk. And this applies to all faculty, whether or not they happen to be members of the IRB.

The role of Ross Woolley on the IRB and in his contacts with the heart team and the patient have been discussed, both by Dr. Renée Fox and by Dr. Altman. From my observations, Dr. Woolley's role developed and grew as the heart experiment progressed. Perhaps we were remiss in failing to define the role of all IRB members prior to the experiment. We thought we had. But all events are not foreseeable. Medicine, more than law, for instance, is a participatory process. As you make one decision it will affect future ones. Prescribing digitalis is an example. You cannot decide today how much you will prescribe tomorrow until you evaluate the effects of today's dosage. Therefore, I don't think we should be critical of ourselves for not having all of the answers to all of the questions before we started the experiment. We must engage in the process to some extent and then ask you and the public to judge whether or not we had made sufficient preparations.

Back to Ross Woolley. In addition to his role as an IRB member who votes on issues, he began a second role—to act as monitor for the IRB subcommittee on the artificial heart program. It was only natural that he began to assume greater importance to Bill DeVries because Bill could check with Ross to be certain that nothing he was doing was exceeding IRB guidelines. This is my opinion and not Bill's. Bill felt reassured by his frequent contacts with Ross, and he asked Ross to play an increasingly important role in monitoring this process on a regular basis. Larry Altman asked whether Ross was protecting the patient, the institution, or the IRB. It seems to me that those were all part of the same process. It was important that there be no conflict of interest among the three or conditions would deteriorate. Ross was there to see that the surgeons' enthusiasm for the success of the experiment did not, in any way, endanger or compromise the patient. He was also attempting to determine that the spirit as well as the letter of the IRB's approval was being carried out.

Now if Ross or Bill or I tell reporters, in response to a question, that they are not privileged to see Barney's medical record, even though it is several months after his death, one could interpret that to be in self-interest, in the interest of the patient, or in the interest of the university and hospital. It doesn't really matter. But it is important that the correct decision is made not to release the medical record.

COMMERCIALISM

Concerning your question, Larry, about whether there is an embargo on scientific publications because of a clause in the *Reader's Digest* contract with the Clark family, the answer is no. Any professional publications may be printed immediately. The proceedings of this conference may be published tomorrow if Marge Shaw can finish editing by that time. The chapters Renée Fox and Judith Swazey have written for their book can appear any time they choose because there is no connection between professional publications and the *Reader's Digest* contract.

Whether or not the Clarks could pay the hospital bill is unrelated to their liberty to strike a deal with *Reader's Digest* or anyone else. Mrs. Clark could be a millionaire or a pauper, and it would not affect her right to enter into a contract. She could sell the whole story or parts of the story, at her own choosing. This is not related to her poverty, her affluence, or her outstanding bills. It took us a long time to work through that decision but, quite frankly, it seems to me that that is very clear.

You are quite correct that the hospital bill was the Clark family's responsibility and that was agreed upon before surgery and included in the IRB consent form (see appendix A, section 17). But we came to feel that they were making an enormous contribution to science, and, frankly, the concept of family that Dr. Fox discussed was growing among us. So I looked for private monies, not tax funds or state funds, but funds that had been given to the University of Utah for discretionary use. We found such monies, and we are still receiving donations from private citizens. Medicare paid a portion of the bill.

I went to Mrs. Clark in January and said, "Mrs. Clark, the university has found a way to pay the bill." (All physician charges were waived in advance and the Clarks were told so.) This offer by the university had no relationship to checkbook journalism. It was not tied to an infringement of their rights to sell all or part of their story. We had a hard time working through all of this, but we feel satisfied now and we plan to make it clear from the very beginning in the next experimental case that there will be no patient contributions required.

Regarding the query about the videotape of the operation, there has been no holdup on its release to the public because of the contract with *Reader's Digest*. Again, the two issues are unrelated. Mrs. Clark is not comfortable with the release of the tape at this time. It has been argued that we should ignore Mrs. Clark's views on this matter and release the tape anyway. Our university educational station has produced a good documentary and would like to show it to the world. But Bill and I have promised Mrs. Clark that until she is ready, it will not be released. They are modifying the film from time to time, and they may arrive at a compromise with her so that she and her family would be comfortable with its release.

With respect to Kolff Medical, we are very proud of the fact that the university initiates spin-offs from its research to commercial operations. A university is not a good place to build gadgets; it is not a good manufacturing company. Thus, when an invention reaches the point of commercial manufacture, it is better to sell the patent or release licenses to private industry. Other universities have done the same thing. So Kolff Medical has spun off from its university ties. In the process, it has given the university a modest amount of stock. I think it is 5 percent, which is a usual figure. This is not different from the arrangements made elsewhere for the royalties on vitamin D or on warfarin, an anticoagulant. The royalties returned to the universities are generally used to fund more research, and we expect to use our royalties that way, if Kolff Medical makes some profit in the future.

Is there a conflict of interest if the university is supporting a heart project and also has a 5 percent interest in a company that, if it prospers because its products are used in the project, will bring money to the university? Yes, there is a conflict of interest, but it is a very modest one. And it is one that is clearly declared and announced to the public so that people can make their own judgments about the degree of conflict. But it is no different, in my estimation, than the conflict between Wisconsin and vitamin D or between the University of California at San Francisco and genetic engineering.

Do university employees own stock in Kolff Medical? Yes, some do, but we are very careful to determine that no one who has any clinical discretion or makes clinical decisions on the artificial heart team has any Kolff stock. It is important to clearly separate these two types of individuals. Rob Jarvik has stock in Kolff Medical and he has a part-time adjunct appointment with the university for which he is compensated $10,000 for 20 percent time. Dr. Donald Olsen, the veterinary surgeon in the animal barn, also holds Kolff Medical stock. But they make no discretionary judgments with respect to patients or their care. No one who will be making judgments about whether the artificial heart program is going to proceed or cease has a financial interest in Kolff Medical.[3]

Now I suspect that the university's relationship with Kolff Medical is not yet perfected. It may never be perfect, and your criticisms are invited. We will certainly discuss it openly, and write about it in the future. Many universities are coping with the problem of university-governmental-industrial relationships; these are new and unfamiliar territories for many of us, and we are trying to find the best arrangement that will be both fair and free from conflict of interest. This issue is especially important for state-supported universities. I hope that a year from now our arrangements will be better defined.

Regarding the question about the broken valve, we have given the university IRB a full report and disclosure, and I think that is where the report should be made. Whether or not there would be anxiety raised in other candidates if they knew the identity of the manufacturer of the broken valve is a difficult thing to judge. It is more important to know the cause of the break and how to prevent it from happening again than to know the name of the manufacturer, and that is what we have been studying.

THE NASA ANALOGY

I don't think I ever meant to say that our reporting was analogous to that of NASA but rather that the analogy referred to commercial journalism. I was interested in reading *The Right Stuff*, which reminded me of something I had forgotten: the astronauts sold their story to *Life* for $50,000, I believe. That was the analogy I meant to make. No one at the university has sold his or her story but, as reported, the Clark family sold its story to *Reader's Digest*.

NAMING THE MODELS OF THE ARTIFICIAL HEART

We have never hidden from the public an understanding of the development of various models of the artificial heart. Perhaps we were remiss in failing to outline to the press, in greater detail, the historical development of each model. We had a fire in the old building that housed the artificial organ program six or seven years ago, and many of the older models were burned. They had been on display before the fire. *Life* carried a pictorial review of all of the old models and that article was available two or three years ago.

I can acknowledge the dispute over priorities in the development of various models of the artificial heart. Dr. Clifford Kwan-Gett believes that he did not receive proper credit for his contributions to the program. So I asked Pam Fogel for a history of the devices. Dr. Kolff wrote the history, Pam edited it, and it was released. However, Kwan-Gett is still not satisfied. Maybe he is right, but we don't know. So we set up a panel of independent people headed by Dr. James Brophy to review all of the evidence that we can amass to see who deserves credit for each piece of the research and development—ideas, design, engineering, and other contributions.

THE SECOND CASE

Larry is correct in that Dr. Lyle Joyce has left the university and has gone to Minnesota. He wanted to stay and participate in the second implant, but it has been delayed so long that he finally took an offer that was available to him in Minneapolis. He has promised to return when he is needed by Bill DeVries, and his partners in his new venture have agreed to this arrangement.

Well, there are the answers to your questions, Larry. I may have missed some, but I think we do have answers to most of the questions that you raised. Yours were searching, vigorous questions that consultants should expose us to, and I believe that this is just the type of exchange that Margery Shaw and I had in mind when we planned this conference. I really think that the university has nothing to fear from criticism as long as we make reasonable plans and report accurately. I would argue that we made reasonable and good plans for the heart project. And our plans are continuing. As long as we remain alert and can learn things from the experiment and from feedback from others, we are doing the best we can. We must also constantly remind ourselves that, although self-confidence is a necessary ingredient of any experiment, we don't know everything and we will not supply answers prematurely. We must continue to probe and question in order to get accurate answers. So thank you, Larry, for your provocative and challenging questions, and thank you for your friendship.

NOTES

    1. The article was published in February 1984: William C. DeVries, Jeffrey L. Anderson, Lyle D. Joyce, Fred L. Anderson, Elizabeth H. Hammond, Robert K. Jarvik, and Willem J. Kolff, "Clinical Use of the Total Artificial Heart," *New England Journal of Medicine* 310 (2 February 1984): 273–78.
    2. William C. DeVries and Lyle D. Joyce, "The Implantation of the Total Artificial Heart for the Treatment of Endstage Cardiomyopathy," *Journal of Thoracic and Cardiovascular Surgery*, in press.
    3. Dr. Robert Jarvik interrupted to make an important point about Dr. Kolff's and others' reluctance to discuss any aspect of Kolff Medical with the press or with any other party. They were bound by Securities and Exchange Commission regulations to refrain from publicly discussing any business aspects of the corporation that might affect stock price until ninety days after the public offering. The ninety days ended on the second day of the conference.

Deliberations of the Utah Institutional Review Board Concerning the Artificial Heart

JOHN A. BOSSO

INTRODUCTION

Institutional review boards (IRBS) are charged with the task of protecting the rights and welfare of human research subjects. Although the mandate for this responsibility originates from the Department of Health and Human Services, it is applied locally by IRBS in hospitals and medical centers. IRBS apply the federal regulations[1] according to their own interpretation and locally developed policies and procedures to research involving human subjects that is financially supported by the federal government and often to all research regardless of the funding source. The interpretation and application of these regulations by the University of Utah Institutional Review Board for Research with Human Subjects have been described elsewhere.[2] In carrying out its charge to protect human subjects, an IRB performs two basic functions. The first is to assure that the potential benefits to the research subject outweigh the potential risks that may occur through participation. Second, the IRB must assure that an adequate informed consent process is provided. In carrying out these procedures, other issues such as confidentiality, methods of subject recruitment and selection, and handling of medical records are also addressed.

THE HISTORY OF IRB ACTIONS CONCERNING THE ARTIFICIAL HEART PROTOCOL

The first artificial heart implantation research protocol was received for consideration by the University of Utah IRB in October of 1980. After an agreement was reached with the investigators to limit the potential subject population to those patients whose hearts cease during cardiac surgery and cannot be restarted, and after significant revision of the consent form, this protocol was approved in February of 1981. In the following year, several patients agreed to implantation of the artificial heart under these circumstances, but since no complications arose in the treatment of these consenting subjects, no implant operations were performed. The investigators subsequently requested that the prospective recipient pool be expanded to include patients with cardiomyopathy who were in Class IV congestive failure for at least eight weeks, as defined by the New York State Heart Association: "Class IV patients have the inability to carry on any physical activity without discomfort. Symptoms of discomfort are present even at rest. With any physical activity, increased discomfort is experienced." Such patients were to be in such a state that no other forms of therapy, short of heart replacement (human heart transplantation or artificial heart implantation) were tenable. A protocol for implantation of the artificial heart in cardiomyopathy patients was approved in May of 1982. In December of 1982, Dr. Barney Clark became the first recipient of this device under the Utah cardiomyopathy protocol.

An IRB monitor was assigned to observe the investigative team to ensure that the informed consent process and research protocol agreed upon were adhered to. This assignment was significantly expanded by the monitor without the knowledge of the IRB and will be discussed later.

The first patient, Dr. Barney Clark, died 112 days after implantation. A subcommittee of the IRB was formed in January of 1983 to gather information about this first case that could be applied to the benefit-risk and informed consent considerations of the board for future cases. The subcommittee gathered such information largely by interviewing individuals involved with the first case, including the investigators. A subcommittee report to the entire IRB was generated and submitted in May of 1983. This report pointed out possible shortcomings with the first case, made recommendations for changes in the protocol, and raised a number of questions to be answered by the investigative team. One of the questions was how complications, such as those encountered with the first case, would be handled in subsequent cases. This report was received and considered but not accepted by the IRB because it left a number of questions unanswered. These included a description of how the first subject was selected, a statement of new research questions to be answered by subsequent cases (in addition to original questions), and a list of problems encountered with the first case and how they were handled. Through a series of communications and meetings with the principal investigator, it was agreed that a full, detailed report of the first case should be submitted for full IRB review along with a revised protocol and consent form.

ONGOING CONCERNS OF THE IRB ABOUT THE ARTIFICIAL HEART

At some point in medical research of this type, research in applicable animal models is exhausted and research in human subjects is begun. An obvious question for an IRB in these instances is whether the device, procedure, or drug has been adequately evaluated in animals to assure an acceptable level of safety for experimental application in humans. Whether this point has been reached with the artificial heart has been a continuing question of the IRB. The answer to this question lies in the results of the first few implantations in humans, and it is through careful review of this experience that the IRB will reach its conclusions. The criteria for and selection process of the most appropriate experimental subject have been and continue to be a concern of the IRB and the research investigators. Naturally, a healthy adult would be a positive proving ground for the artificial heart, but such a selection is obviously inappropriate from ethical and societal perspectives. On the other end of the spectrum is the individual who is terminally ill, so ill that the heart replacement represents the sole means of survival. Such patients often have multiple organ systems so compromised that they provide little or limited potential for successful improvement of their clinical condition. New York State Heart Association Class IV patients often fall in this category. Nonetheless, this was the category of patients approved as recipients under the cardiomyopathy protocol. It may well be that other cardiomyopathy patients who have been in Class IV for a shorter period of time than the Food and Drug Administration–approved minimum of eight weeks are more appropriate candidates.

Designing an adequate informed consent form and deciding on protocols for the consent process for the artificial heart research endeavor has been a complicated task in which the IRB has assisted the investigators. The result was an eleven-page written consent form. A lengthy consent form is cumbersome and may be confusing. Reading and understanding such a form is obviously a formidable task. At the same time, full disclosure of experimental procedures, potential risks and benefits, and other information relevant to participation in research is a requirement under federal regulations. It is well understood, however, that a written consent form only represents part of the informed consent process and that verbal communication between the investigator and the potential research subject is more important and perhaps more effective than any written document.

The quality of life that can be reasonably expected after implantation of an artificial heart has been an area of vigorous debate. Although this concept may be defined or quantified by the various investigators or the IRB, it is really the patient who must identify what is a suitable quality of life. We must not lose sight of that concept. It is therefore vital that the potential subject be informed of what life may be expected to be like once the artificial heart is implanted.

REFLECTIONS ON CRITICISMS OF THE IRB

The IRB has been criticized for the length of time it is taking to reapprove the artificial heart protocol subsequent to the conclusion of the first case. A number of reasons account for this delay.

The original considerations of the IRB concerning risk versus benefit and informed consent were based on suppositions and hypotheses because it had to extrapolate from animal experiments to what might occur in humans. Therefore, it was believed to be vital that these issues be reassessed based on experience and knowledge gained through the first case. A subcommittee was formed to gather this information and report to the full IRB with its findings and recommendations. The subcommittee took several months to complete this task. Its final report was considered to be incomplete by the IRB, however, largely because the full, written report on the first case had not been received from the investigators. Because of this, all of the information needed by the IRB for its risk-benefit analysis was not yet available. Subsequent IRB deliberations generated a request for more information from the investigators. However, written requests to the principal investigator were ineffectual because of lack of clarity regarding desired format and detail. An IRB meeting was held with the principal investigator to discuss this problem and clarify the committee's needs.[3] It is obvious, in retrospect, that the IRB was inefficient in making its needs clear to the investigators and in its collection of desired information. Lessons have been learned that should help expedite this process after the next implant.

Dr. Larry Altman and others have commented on the differences among procedures used by the Utah IRB and those of other IRBs across the nation. Altman has also asked whether the Utah IRB is attempting to protect the experimental subject or the institution.

The Utah IRB operates under the same federal regulations that all IRBs do. The only room for variation is in the interpretation of those regulations (where intent is not totally clear) and in the vigor in which they are applied. As the Utah IRB takes its responsibilities very seriously, it may be that it applies the federal regulations more rigorously than do other IRBs. The IRB is clearly charged with the protection of the rights and welfare of experimental research subjects. Any notion to the contrary is without basis. It should be noted, however, that an IRB that conscientiously carries out its charge secondarily protects the institution through the prevention of unethical or unsound research that may result in criticism or even litigation. This secondary benefit (to the institution), however, is never the primary concern of the IRB and never should be. At most, it is a positive fallout of ethical concerns for the patient-subjects.

Dr. Altman also raised the issue of accountability of the Utah IRB. An IRB is accountable to its parent institution, which has assured the Department of Health and Human Services that its regulations regarding research in human subjects will be followed. However, the IRB satisfies its responsibility to the institution by carrying out its assigned functions. The results of IRB deliberations, approvals, and disapprovals for proposed studies, are another matter. An IRB, if appropriately carrying out its task according to the federal regulations, is not accountable for its actions to the institution or to the investigator. As long as an IRB conforms to federal regulations, it represents an autonomous body. It could be argued that IRBs are, in a sense, accountable to the general public. It is recognized, however, that this is a philosophical stance and that the general public has no obvious route of input to an IRB except through lay representatives on the committee.

As mentioned earlier, the role of the individual assigned by the IRB to monitor ethical issues arising during the first implant grew beyond the board's intent. The individual involved was drawn by both professional interest and personal concern into a position in which it was difficult to distinguish him as an IRB monitor or as a member of the investigative team. It is not surprising that questions of conflict of interest arose. While no conflict of interest could be demonstrated, the monitor's role developed into something neither envisioned nor desired by the IRB. The monitor's role has subsequently been redefined and in the future will be limited to observation of the consent process.

In September of 1983, the minutes of one of several previous IRB meetings concerning the artificial heart were leaked to local news media by a person or persons who remain unknown. Excerpts from these minutes were subsequently aired on local and national news programs. Because these excerpts were presented out of context their impact was misleading. Among other inaccuracies was the contention that the IRB has determined that the first artificial heart recipient did not meet the inclusion criteria of the research protocol. In reality, the minutes of that particular meeting reflected the fact that the IRB did not yet have all the information it needed to conclude its deliberations. No conclusions regarding the first case had been reached. This misrepresentation of IRB deliberations resulted in considerable consternation for IRB members, the investigators, the family of the first recipient, and other individuals involved in the first case.

The IRB was quite concerned that its confidential minutes had become public information. It believed that this would compromise further IRB deliberations, which had always been held in a free forum in which members could express views and ask questions in an uninhibited manner. Such a forum is felt to be vital to the IRB's appropriately carrying out its responsibilities. An inhibiting environment could cause members to be very careful about what they said and perhaps even prevent the raising of certain issues.

As the perpetrator of this event was never identified, the IRB took several resultant actions. The IRB policies and procedures were rewritten to stress the fact that all IRB minutes are confidential and should not be shared outside the board. The manner of recording minutes was changed so that no direct quotes are recorded and specific speakers are not identified. This is, of course, a sad state of affairs, but it has been effective in maintaining frank discussions in the meetings. Dr. Altman has suggested that the IRB set itself up for this occurrence by being so secretive about its proceedings. To counter this possibility, the IRB has been issuing press releases to keep the media informed of its progress with the artificial heart protocol; however, meetings are still held in strict confidence.

PHILOSOPHY OF THE IRB CONCEPT

What an IRB is, what it does, and what its purpose is seems to be largely unknown or misunderstood in many quarters. Investigators often view IRBs as impediments to research that tie them up with red tape and paperwork. The Utah IRB has often been portrayed in the media in much the same light. It has been suggested that IRBS were originally created because medical investigators could not be trusted to bridle their own enthusiasm for research and to keep the

best interests of their research subjects in mind. IRBs would therefore be expected to provide the appropriate governance. On the other
hand, IRBs do not control or govern medical scientists but instead
assist them in becoming aware of optimal ways to protect the rights
and welfare of research subjects.

Finally, it is appropriate to examine the membership composition of IRBs. Such membership is largely composed of medical scientists who are, themselves, researchers. Thus, it may be suggested
that IRBs and medical scientists are not two distinct groups but are
one and the same. It follows, therefore, that IRBs represent a group
(i.e., medical scientists) that governs itself. Obviously, this is not
completely true, however, because a number of nonscientists and
nonmedical scientists are members of the Utah IRB. It may be argued
that the regulations that IRBs apply were prepared by an outside body
(i.e., the federal government), but it should be recognized that the
medical science community has significant input into their design
and content.

NOTES

1. Protection of Human Subjects, 45 C.F.R. §46 (1983).
2. J. A. Bosso, "The Role of the Institutional Review Board in Research
Involving Human Subjects," *Drug Intelligence and Clinical Pharmacy* 17
(1983): 828–34.
3. By late November 1983 all requested information and a revised protocol and consent form were received and were under active consideration.
The Utah IRB approved these documents and granted permission for a second implant in January 1984. The FDA gave its approval in June 1984. [Note
added on proof.—Ed.]

PART FOUR

Economic, Historical, and Scientific Issues

The Artificial Heart as an Economic Issue

DAVID BLUMENTHAL AND
RICHARD J. ZECKHAUSER

Economic issues have become central to debates about medical technologies and the functioning of our health care system generally. Only recently, under the relentless pressure of rising expenditures, has our society confronted the reality of scarcity in the health care field. This recognition, in turn, has heightened interest in efficiency: making sure that an individual or society gets its money's worth and maximum value from the dollars spent, whether the expenditure is for prenatal care, hospital stays, or new technologies such as the artificial heart. It is efficient expenditures that most of us—physicians, economists, policymakers, consumers, and taxpayers—are after. Even large expenditures well spent are justified and appropriate. The central challenge is defining what is meant by "well spent."

The artificial heart presents this challenge in a particularly poignant and pressing form. Although it resembles other costly medical innovations in many respects, this device has a number of salient special properties. The heart has a unique place in our pantheon of potentially replaceable organs. Throughout history it has been viewed as the physical and symbolic home of quintessential human properties: emotion, spirit, compassion, vitality. And no organ seems more essential to the maintenance of biological life, particularly to the public. Kidney or liver failure may drag on for days or weeks before death ensues. When the heart stops, death is virtually instantaneous.

The cost of providing artificial hearts could also exceed that of treating organ failure of other types or through other means. Many organs—the kidney, liver, heart, lung, and pancreas—can be successfully transplanted. But the availability of donor organs will always limit the use and costs of organ transplantation.[1] The artificial heart faces no such constraint on supply. More hearts can always be produced at the factory. The costs of an individual device and its implantation are high, estimated at $28,000 by Lubeck and Bunker.[2] And the number of potential recipients of this particular technology is as great as for any other organ and perhaps greater. Some 684,000 Americans die of heart disease each year, more than from any other cause. Of course, not all of these people would be candidates to receive an artificial heart. Under restrictive assumptions, the number of possible recipients has been estimated by Lubeck and Bunker at between 16,000 and 66,000. If we include patients over age 65 and with coexistent illnesses (not unreasonable given the history of the end-stage renal disease program), the number of potential recipients could easily exceed 100,000 annually.

Because of its symbolic value, its life-giving potential, and its daunting potential costs, the artificial heart epitomizes the trade-offs inherent in extending life through extraordinary means. It thus threatens the cherished myth that in our society no price is too high to save an identified life.[3] This myth is valuable and comforting. In the past, we have paid heavily to preserve it. The end-stage renal disease program and the spread of third-party coverage for organ transplantation are examples.[4] The artificial heart, however, may prove to be the first instance in which the growing realization that cost significantly exceeds benefit forces us to limit or prohibit the use of a technology even though an identifiable group of patients may die as a result. The price of preserving the myth that life is priceless may prove too high.

Economists have codified two major commonsense approaches to such wrenching decisions. First, the *economics of governance* clarifies the effects of the organization and financing of our health care system on the efficiency with which we use scarce resources, such as those necessary to produce, install, and maintain the artificial heart. Understanding such relationships enriches the range of alternatives available to policymakers struggling to protect human values while limiting costs. Second, the *economics of project selection* provides tools for thinking about the relative values of alternative projects, like the artificial heart, and for deciding which should be undertaken, which should be dropped, and which should be postponed.

In a moment, we will comment on how each of these two approaches contributes to the debate about the artificial heart. Before proceeding, however, a few words of caution are in order. To begin with, economics yields no magical key to ethical insight. Indeed, economists usually claim not even to compete in that arena, for they believe that the tools they apply are largely value free. Economics does remind us, however, that decision makers should pay close attention to how consumers themselves value a good, as revealed by price in market transactions, and that public decision makers should worry about how their constituencies feel about (i.e., value the consequences of) the choices at hand. Alas, the market does not reveal what individuals would pay for artificial hearts; even goods offering distant parallels are hard to find. This leads to another cautionary word.

Economic analysis has distinct limitations when confronting health care problems. Two of these limitations, discussed in more detail below, are (*a*) the difficulty of measuring the output of health care investments and (*b*) the fact that health care markets depart in so many respects from the ideal of the competitive marketplace, the area in which the economist's measuring rod, price, is the most accurate indicator of value. Nevertheless, we would argue that economic reasoning can improve on unaided intuition in enabling us to decide how to use health care resources most efficiently. In fact, economics often makes its greatest contribution in precisely those situations in which the goods (like health care) are difficult to value and normal markets do not exist. In such areas, the bureaucrat's unaided intuition or the tug and haul of the political process is most likely to go far astray. If the question were whether to buy or produce carrots or apples, economics would have relatively little to contribute. Consumers, farmers, and government officials could be expected to make efficient decisions on their own.

THE ECONOMICS OF GOVERNANCE

As most are aware, an influential group of economists, enamored of the competitive model, has made a powerful case in recent years for fundamental reforms in the governance of our health care system. Those reforms contain an implicit answer to the question of whether we should develop the artificial heart. The argument, very briefly, is as follows.

The theory of welfare economics holds that if certain assumptions are met concerning the nature of a particular economic sector, then free competition produces an optimal distribution of goods and services, resources are used as efficiently as possible, and consumer welfare is maximized in the sense that no individual can be made better off without making someone else worse off. Economists have noted that the spread of health insurance coverage, fostered by federal subsidies, has seriously undermined the ability of our health care system to function as a competitive market.[5,6] Protected by insurance, which itself is purchased at a discount, consumers do not encounter effective prices (that is, they pay at most a fraction of the cost) when buying health care services, and producers need not compete for customers on the basis of cost. Too much health care is bought, and production tends to be inefficient and overpriced.

Recognizing that the present health care market has peculiar features that render classic models of competition unsuitable, advocates of increased price competition have developed schemes to reform the health care system to approximate the conditions assumed by the theory of welfare economics. By eliminating tax subsidies for the purchase of insurance and by requiring employers to offer employees a choice among insurance options, these proposals attempt to foster competition among alternative health care plans, including health maintenance organizations. The competition, it is hoped, would result in a more efficient use of resources and in the provision of health services in a manner more responsive to consumer choice.

How would such reforms in the organization and financing of the health care system help us with the problem of the artificial heart? Some consumers will purchase the right to have an artificial heart (if needed) by joining insurance plans that provide it as a covered benefit. The price of the coverage may be substantial. But if consumers do not consider the artificial heart worth the price charged by the insurance plan, then they will not purchase coverage for it, manufacturers will not find a market, and the innovation will wither. Thus, decentralized consumer decisions, rather than governmental decree, would guide the fate of the artificial heart.[7]

Some may object on ethical grounds to treating health care as just another consumer item, whose availability and distribution would depend on market forces.[8] Others may doubt that procompetitive proposals could be implemented and function as proposed.[9] Our purpose here is not to evaluate the merits of any particular plan or to prescribe an optimal structure for our health care system. Nor do we mean to imply that systemic change is the only answer to the question of whether and how to proceed with developing the artificial heart. Rather, we wish to highlight three points.

First, the organization and financing of the health care system should not be ignored in discussing the artificial heart. We have argued elsewhere that the inappropriate or excessive use of health care technologies is frequently the symptom of more fundamental maladies in our health care system, notably financial malincentives that promote the use of services without sufficient attention to their marginal costs.[10] An adequate solution to our problems with the artificial heart may depend on correcting those malincentives, whether through procompetitive reforms or other modifications in third-party reimbursement rules. Indeed, if we fail to address fundamental problems in the organization and financing of our health care system, we are almost certain to be dissatisfied with the way the artificial heart is distributed and used, should it become available.

Second, this technology should not be employed as a stalking-horse for disagreements about other more fundamental issues related to the way our health care system is governed. Some may favor the artificial heart because they believe that, once it is available, its expense will strengthen the moral and political case for national health insurance. Others may oppose it for precisely the same reason, arguing that universal entitlement results in excessive consumption of health care services relative to other goods and services. The point is not that either case is right or wrong but that the proponents for both seem primarily concerned with the governance of the health care system, not the artificial heart. We must make clear our agendas. Only then can the technology itself get a fair and thorough appraisal.

Third, we must be realistic about likely reforms in the health care system. Though we would argue strenuously for such reforms as part of any strategy our society adopts toward the artificial heart, we cannot assert confidently that meaningful or beneficial changes will be implemented before the artificial heart—or its more modest cousin the left ventricular assist device—becomes widely available. In the short term, therefore, policymakers must decide whether and how to develop the artificial heart in the context of our current health care system: a system that, though changing, incorporates widespread, though unequal, insurance against the cost of illness and few incentives for restraint in the use of expensive health care resources. Under these circumstances, we feel the looming costs of this new technology may create strong pressures for regulatory action to limit or proscribe its use. Any such decision should be made on the basis of the best possible analysis of the costs and benefits of this new medical device in the ways it is likely to be used. Economics provides tools for such an analysis, though, as we shall see, those tools may not yield definitive answers.

THE ECONOMICS OF PROJECT SELECTION

Research and Development

One of the first issues confronting policymakers, and especially federal research administrators, is whether to continue supporting research and development related to the artificial heart. Federal authorities have already invested roughly $180 million over the last seventeen years for research and development related to this new device, and public support continues at a rate of about $10 million annually.[11] Should society continue this investment?

Continued investment in research and development projects is often justified on the grounds that so much has already been committed that it would be absurd to stop now. The fallacy of that view is elegantly summarized in the common aphorism "Don't throw good money after bad." Society should be concerned with the return on investment of marginal dollars, not with the sunk costs of a project. If the artificial heart is not going to yield an adequate return on additional investments in research and development, such expenditures only compound past mistakes.

A more appropriate rule to guide decisions about whether to proceed with research and development is the following: don't invest further unless the sum of discounted future expected consumers' and producers' surplus will equal the additional costs of your research and development program. In other words, don't undertake further artificial heart research unless, on average, you expect to get back your value in benefits to patients and manufacturers of the device. We might call this the "rational" model for choosing (and choosing whether to continue) research and development projects.[12]

We will comment shortly on the difficulties in applying cost-benefit analysis and cost-effectiveness analysis to developed health care technologies. For now, we note that assessing benefits and costs for research and development projects is substantially more hazardous. The reason, not surprisingly, is that the uncertainties about both the costs and the benefits of a research and development investment are considerably greater than those for a more developed and tested technology. The artificial heart must still overcome major problems related to the development of an adequate portable power source. This may take many more years and dollars than expected. Alternatively, unanticipated breakthroughs may dramatically alter the costs of the device, the difficulties of implanting it, and the long-term benefits for patients. Certainly, we cannot assume that the artificial heart that becomes commercially available on a large scale will be anything like the cumbersome and confining device that sustained Barney Clark for 112 days.

In predicting the value of research and development investments, further uncertainties surround the possibility of important spin-offs unrelated to the purpose of the project. The National Cancer Institute's heavy investment in isolating a viral cause of cancer was widely criticized in the mid-1970s when it appeared unlikely to result in clinically useful results. However, funds for virologic research supported David Baltimore's Nobel Prize–winning work and helped to speed the development of recombinant DNA technology, whose potential benefits in oncology and other fields are awesome. Some of the most important results of human experimentation with the artificial heart may stem from improvements in our understanding of cardiovascular physiology as recipients are monitored.

Uncertainties in calculating the expected value or cost of a research and development investment—whether for the artificial heart or other projects—argue for considering another model in deciding whether to fund research and development ventures. We might call this the "quasi-rational" model. If the costs of the proposed research are small and the potential benefits comparatively large (though uncertain), then proceed. Little is lost and gains may be huge. If the research does not pay off or if the costs of using the developed product are found to outweigh the benefits, then the research may be halted at a later stage or the product shelved.

This model acknowledges that fine calculations of cost and benefit may be impossible at early stages of project development. The solution is to risk small amounts of resources, provided large gains are possible, and to allow for the possibility of gathering more information before making final decisions about the value of the project.[13] Quite simply, this strategy amounts to paying for information. Learning narrows uncertainty. Applied to the artificial heart, this model might suggest that $10 million a year is relatively little to pay for a device that may turn out to extend meaningful life by a substantial number of years for tens of thousands of individuals. If the benefits of the device are smaller than anticipated or if the costs of its manufacture, implantation, and maintenance prove to be too great in comparison with the benefits, we can decide to forego its use at an appropriate future time.

If the artificial heart, once developed, were priced on the basis of its marginal cost, the quasi-rational model for deciding about the current research and development investment would be compelling. But the reality is that virtually no one would pay for his or her own artificial heart. Expenses would be covered by private insurance or the government. There would be no effective limit on demand. Thus, once a technology like the artificial heart is sufficiently developed to be used, its spread may be almost impossible to contain under our current health care system. Even if we learn a substantial amount about the costs and benefits of the artificial heart, we may not make appropriate decisions down the line. In particular, we may find ourselves making the device widely available despite the fact that its costs substantially exceed its benefits.

Because of its potential cost, the artificial heart may prove an exception to the pattern that available life-saving technologies become entitlements to those who need them. If not, the expenditures could be staggering. This possibility creates strong pressure to scrutinize the device at the stage of research and development, even though the tools of rational analysis may be difficult to apply and some decisions must be expected to prove faulty. We might call this "the last-secure-stopping-point" argument for assessing and possibly curtailing technologies at the research and development stage.[14]

To buttress the case for such early intervention in the creation of new health care technologies, Sapolsky draws an interesting contrast between research and development for health care and for the military, another sector in which small governmental expenditures for research and development often balloon into multibillion dollar procurement programs.[15] Sapolsky points out that in setting budgets for research and development on such programs as the MX missile or the Trident submarine, deployment costs are a major issue. Such concerns are seldom raised with respect to research on health care devices. Weinstein argues convincingly that cost-effectiveness and decision analysis can assist in setting priorities for research concerning preventable causes of cancer.[16]

An attempt to balance these arguments about whether and how to make decisions concerning the funding of research and development on health care technologies suggests the following position: given the realities of our health care system, it may prove desirable to slow or to discontinue federal support of certain applied research projects because it appears that the costs of finished products will substantially outweigh the benefits. But if this approach is employed, the following qualifications and concerns should be kept in mind.

First, cost-effectiveness analysis or cost-benefit analysis should be only one of many yardsticks applied in making such choices. Other considerations should include the political appeal of particular projects and their ethical, social, and legal implications. Second, although it may be appropriate to apply cost-benefit analysis, cost-effectiveness analysis, or both to highly applied research projects (like the Trident missile or testing chemical carcinogens), these tools have relatively little to offer in assessing more basic research endeavors, such as work on fundamental properties of living organisms or basic mechanisms of disease. Third, in the case of the artificial heart, as well as in most other applied research projects, the information necessary to compare a particular use of research and development funds with alternative uses does not exist. This limits our ability to make reasonable decisions about the relative merits of research and development projects in the health field. Fourth, given the absence of concrete relevant data, we must be sensitive to the danger that prejudice rather than careful analysis will determine whether we proceed with particular research and development projects.

The potential difficulties that we face in accurately assessing the value of research and development projects provide a strong argument for making reforms in the health care system that would permit the use of the quasi-rational approach to allocating research and development dollars. If we were more confident of our ability to halt a project like the artificial heart once it became available (assuming that its costs were then expected to exceed its benefits substantially) and if our system embodied more appropriate financial incentives concerning the use of health care technologies, then we could be far more relaxed and permissive in our treatment of research and development projects. This strikes us as a more satisfactory approach to the allocation of research and development funds than early curtailments on the basis of speculation.

Before leaving the subject of research on the artificial heart, we wish to comment briefly on the commonly made assertion that the federal government's past and continuing investment in this effort constitutes a strong justification for making the heart equally available to all members of our society. Given the staggering cost of the artificial heart, this implies a governmental obligation to subsidize all or part of the cost of providing the device for the great bulk of potential recipients. There may be an ethical or legal case for this viewpoint; however, the economic argument is tenuous at best. For classic reasons of market failure, private interests tend to underinvest in research and development activities in a competitive market. Many analysts, therefore, feel comfortable with government support of research and development activities in health and in other fields. Overall, such support probably results in greater productivity and more efficient use of existing resources than if the market were left to its own devices. However, in assuming all or part of the marginal costs of products in health or other fields, the government induces consumers to purchase excessive amounts of the good in question. If efficiency in the use of resources is the goal, therefore, government support of research and development makes sense, but government subsidization of the finished products does not.

Even the legal or ethical case for making the artificial heart universally available does not seem to rest principally on the fact of public support of the research and development that created it. To see this, we need only examine our behavior in other fields. Government funds played a critical role in the development of the first electronic computer, the perfection of the semiconductor, and advances in aviation.[17] Few would argue, however, that the federal government is obliged to make personal computers or airline seats universally available. Many of us would wish to distinguish the artificial heart from these other goods. The reason, we would argue, has little to do with governmental support of research and development. Rather, the key factors are our feelings about health care as a special good, our views about the sacredness of life, and our continued unwillingness to permit the death of visible, identifiable patients when there exists a means to prolong their lives.

Cost-benefit and Cost-effectiveness Analysis

It has become axiomatic that cost-benefit analysis, cost-effectiveness analysis, or both should precede decisions on whether and how to use a health care technology. Methods for applying these techniques are well described elsewhere.[18,19] They constitute two valuable approaches to optimizing the use of constrained (i.e., scarce) resources.

Lubeck and Bunker have applied cost-effectiveness analysis to the artificial heart.[20] As all workers in such exercises, they were forced to make a number of assumptions concerning the characteristics and number of potential recipients, the efficacy of the device, and the rate at which patients would consume resources during and after implantation. Although one could quibble with aspects of the analysis, it is the most complete and thorough attempt of which we are aware. Lubeck and Bunker estimate that the availability of the artificial heart could increase the life expectancy of the average twenty-five—year—old American by seven to thirty-five days. For those twenty-five—year—olds destined to die from ischemic heart disease, the device would increase life expectancy by anywhere from 0.13 years to 0.60 years. For actual recipients with ischemic disease, it would extend life expectancy 1.6–3.6 years on average. Estimating implantation costs at $28,000 per patient, follow-up costs at $2,000 a year, and a five-year survival rate similar to that of heart transplants, the authors project annual costs of about $1.1 billion. This calculation assumes that roughly 33,600 patients receive the device annually. Since the model for predicting costs differs from the model for estimating changes in life expectancy, a true cost-effectiveness ratio cannot be calculated from Lubeck and Bunker's work. Nevertheless, these figures indicate that a fully operational program for installing artificial hearts would cost several billions of dollars and would prolong the life of a subset of potential recipients by 1.6 years to 3.6 years.

One of the technical problems with Lubeck and Bunker's work is that in calculating project costs they assume recipients of the artificial heart would have died at the time of implantation if the device had not been installed. Physicians, however, are not so skilled at predicting death that they can select for surgery only those patients on the verge of instant demise, even assuming that they were medically desirable. Some patients chosen to receive the artificial heart would have lived for some time and received expensive medical care even if they had not been given the device. Lubeck and Bunker's estimates of the incremental costs of the artificial heart are, therefore, biased upward.

Such technical issues are more easily resolved than the larger dilemmas facing policymakers who might wish to use cost-benefit and cost-effectiveness analyses for deciding whether and how to pursue the development of the artificial heart or other technologies. Among these less tractable problems, three deserve special mention: measuring health care outputs, dealing with uncertainty, and limited knowledge of the cost-effectiveness of alternative health care investments.

The question of how to measure and value the benefits of health care programs has been widely discussed. Cost-benefit analysis confronts this problem most directly, because it attempts to reduce both costs and benefits to a single metric, usually dollars. This raises troubling and unresolved issues about how to assign dollar values to the years of life gained from health care interventions. A number of techniques are currently used. None is totally satisfying.[21]

Cost-effectiveness analysis skirts the problem of directly valuing life-years by reporting program results in terms of units of benefit (e.g., life-years saved) per dollar of investment. However, cost-effectiveness analysis should still deal with the thorny issue (usually avoided in practice) of how to adjust for effects of health care interventions on quality of life.[22] Failure to consider quality of life—measuring only life-years gained—would obviously lead to a substantial overestimate of the benefits of the artificial heart. (Undoubtedly, the enormous medical and social problems Dr. Clark experienced will be substantially ameliorated as the device improves and physicians gain more experience with its implantation. But even the individual who receives a perfected artificial heart is unlikely to have the same quality of life as a healthy person of the same age.)

Uncertainty complicates the use of cost-benefit and cost-effectiveness analyses. In most analyses of health care technologies, we are uncertain about their current and their future costs and benefits. As noted, these uncertainties are greater for technologies that, like the artificial heart, are early in their developmental life. But even for technologies in more common use, such uncertainties are substantial. Evaluations of heart transplantation, for example, are complicated by uncertainties concerning the long-term survival of transplant patients, by our limited knowledge of the natural history of terminal heart disease, and by uncertainty about how the technique will evolve over time. The introduction of the drug cyclosporine A provides a good illustration of how changes in technologies can affect estimates of their efficacy and costs. This new immunosuppressive agent is estimated to have increased the two-year survival rate of heart transplantation patients at Stanford from 58 percent to 80 percent[23] while reducing the cost by $45,000 per procedure.[24] Another example is the unexpected decline since 1973 in the cost of maintaining an individual patient on dialysis, a result of improvements in the artificial kidney and other factors.

Decision analysis in general, and sensitivity analysis in particular, provides techniques for incorporating such uncertainties into estimating the costs and effectiveness of medical technologies and other investments. Indeed, a major contribution of this array of techniques is to make uncertainty explicit and to force decision makers to grapple with it. We remain convinced, therefore, that decisions taking cost-benefit and cost-effectiveness analyses into account will, on average, prove more satisfactory than those ignoring these approaches. However, as the Office of Technology Assessment has correctly concluded, cost-benefit and cost-effectiveness analyses do not provide quick or simple answers to questions concerning whether to adopt the artificial heart or other technologies.[25]

One other significant difficulty faces decision makers who wish to use cost-effectiveness analysis to assess the merits of the artificial heart. Lubeck and Bunker are almost certainly correct in their conclusion that the artificial heart will fall into that large category of medical investments that are effective at extending life but at considerable cost. For such projects, the decision rule that maximizes the overall effectiveness of resource use is as follows: "rank these projects or technologies in order of increasing cost effectiveness, and adopt them in that order until all resources are used."[26]

In other words, we cannot make rational decisions about the artificial heart in isolation from other competing uses for the resources its development requires. Assume the easiest case, in which monies not spent on the artificial heart would be spent on other health-related projects. Unfortunately, only a tiny fraction of the alternative health care practices, procedures, and programs have been subjected to cost-effectiveness analysis. This drastically limits our ability to make rational decisions about particular projects or indeed about the use of health care resources in general.

Opportunity Costs

A critical issue in health care project selection is the opportunity cost of health care investments—the benefits that might have been realized from alternative uses of invested resources. These foregone benefits, which may or may not equal the price paid for the resources, must be subtracted from program benefits (or added to program costs) to calculate total benefits (or costs) of a health care project.

In health care programs, opportunity costs are important for at least two reasons. First, health care projects like the artificial heart have the potential to use substantial proportions of the available supplies of certain resources, such as cardiac surgeons. This suggests that such projects could affect the market price for such resources. Second, labor markets for the scientists and leading physicians involved in health care programs are thin, especially at the stage of research and development. Moreover, the services of such personnel are not sold on a market basis. As a consequence, their market wage may be a poor indicator of their value to society. For example, it is unlikely that wage differentials among scientists of varying quality will fully reflect differences in their expected productivities. To take an extreme example, Jonas Salk's salary at the time he was developing his vaccine was probably a tiny fraction of the benefits society could expect to receive from his work. Thus, the cost of diverting him to work on another project, say the artificial heart, would have been considerably greater than his wage would indicate. Similarly, the individuals who are now at work developing the artificial heart might be able to make very valuable contributions in other areas, contributions whose dollar values would dwarf the costs of supporting them. An appropriate calculation would look at what they could contribute in their highest valued alternative use, be it improving antipollution technologies, developing artificial limbs, or producing a superior word processor. That quantity is the opportunity cost of having them work on the artificial heart.

The calculation of opportunity costs is complicated by several factors. One is our uncertainty, already discussed at length, concerning the relative cost-effectiveness of alternative health care programs. Lubeck and Bunker explicitly consider the question of opportunity costs and attempt to weigh the value of the artificial heart against the potential expansion of programs for preventing heart disease. They are forced to conclude that "a precise economic comparison of the cost-effectiveness of preventive programs vs. the artificial heart is not feasible until more information is available on the costs, risks and benefits of both approaches."[27]

A second problem in predicting opportunity costs is that the complexities of politics, federal budgets, and the organization of our health care system create uncertainty about where funds for the artificial heart would come from or which programs would benefit if its development were foregone. Two arguments illustrate this point. Advocates of the artificial heart may be tempted to assert that the device could be made available to all potential recipients at the yearly cost of a single nuclear-powered aircraft carrier or fifteen or twenty F-16 fighters. The implication is that the opportunity cost of the artificial heart is the debatable benefits associated with trivial quantities of military hardware. Even if one accepts the view that this incremental military hardware is of little value, the fallacy in the argument is the assumption that the resources used in funding the heart would be drawn from the military budget. If the federal government were to assume the costs of providing artificial hearts, it seems much more likely that funds would be drawn from Medicare, Medicaid, or other health-related programs and from general tax revenues. The result is that these advocates of the artificial heart might dramatically underestimate the opportunity costs associated with it.

Opponents of the artificial heart may be tempted to make another, more plausible argument: the opportunity costs of the artificial heart are high because the program would drain money from critical health initiatives such as biomedical research or disease prevention and health promotion programs.[28] Setting aside our uncertainty concerning the true benefits of these alternative initiatives, the question remains, Will resources not invested in the artificial heart find their way into biomedical research, into smoking cessation programs, into the repair of highways, or into spurring lower taxes?

The answer is not at all straightforward and would require a close examination of the political dynamics of federal health-care budgeting and the manner in which private third-party insurers determine their coverage options. Our own suspicion is that foregoing the artificial heart is unlikely to produce direct increases for biomedical research or smoking cessation programs. However, by increasing pressure on Medicare and Medicaid budgets, pursuing the artificial heart could produce further reductions in benefits for the elderly and the poor and might limit discretionary health programs such as community health centers or maternal and child health programs. An assessment of the opportunity costs of the artificial heart would require a careful evaluation of the distribution and consequences of such cuts. Obviously, the costs associated with such cuts may be just as great as the potential benefits from prevention programs or biomedical research.

Scale of Application

A project's scale or size can affect its attractiveness as an investment. This point may be of consequence for the artificial heart. Increases in the numbers of artificial hearts implanted in this country may increase or decrease its net benefits or costs, depending on a number of considerations. If each additional implantation offered costs and benefits identical to the first, then the more the better. The net benefits of putting in 100,000 would be 100,000 times greater than if only one were implanted. But benefits and costs per implantation may change with scale.

There may be a learning curve or production efficiencies that generate economies of scale. Several factors, however, may cut in the opposite direction, reducing benefits per implantation as numbers increase. As use becomes more widespread, opportunity costs may rise as additional personnel are drawn into the surgical and medical care of patients receiving the device and away from activities in which they were producing greater benefits. More important, the first group of patients may have been ideal candidates, offering the greatest benefits per dollar spent. Later recipients may have more marginal indications; their inclusion will reduce effectiveness/cost ratios.[29]

Finally, if the artificial heart becomes generally available, and if potential recipients are identified, it may be worth undertaking a small number of implantations even if they are less cost-effective than other health care investments. Under such circumstances, the use of the artificial heart might help preserve the valuable myth that life is too sacred to sacrifice, regardless of cost. As the number of devices implanted grows, however, the price of preserving that myth may prove exorbitant.

Implications

On issues ranging from cost per implant to likely effectiveness to the value of alternative uses of the same resources, the uncertainties surrounding the artificial heart are enormous. Given this lack of information and the possibility that the net benefits from the artificial heart could be extraordinary, the authors would not recommend discontinuing the current federal investment in its development. Government support of research and development related to the artificial heart should be reevaluated, however, after the current set of clinical trials. We are rapidly approaching—indeed, we may have already passed—the last secure stopping point for this alluring but extraordinarily expensive technology.

CONCLUSION

The artificial heart, given its symbolic importance and its huge potential costs, may force us to confront directly some choices that we have hitherto evaded. We may now have to decide whether the scarcity of available resources requires that we limit or proscribe the use of a potentially life-prolonging technology. The immediate issue is whether to continue funding research and development on the device, which recently had its first trial in a human being. The decision would be much simpler if our health care system embodied appropriate economic incentives for use of health care technologies. Hence, the best solution to the problem of the artificial heart would include reforms in the governance of our health care system, reforms designed to encourage individual decision-makers, both providers and patients, to consider the costs of any new medical technology when deciding whether it should be used.

Until such fundamental reforms are undertaken, it may be desirable on occasion to slow or discontinue funding of certain medical technologies at the stage of research and development. For the artificial heart, the authors believe, the time to curtail federal support has not yet arrived, though it may be drawing near.

NOTES

1. R. W. Evans, draft of testimony presented at a hearing on organ transplants, U.S. Congress, House, Committee on Energy and Commerce, Subcommittee on Health and the Environment (29 July), 98th Cong., 1st sess., 1983.

2. U.S. Congress, Office of Technology Assessment, *Case Study #9, the Artificial Heart: Costs, Risks, and Benefits*, prepared by D. P. Lubeck and J. P. Bunker (Washington, D.C.: Government Printing Office, 1982).

3. R. J. Zeckhauser, "Coverage for Catastrophic Illness," *Public Policy* 21 (1973): 148–71.

4. American Hospital Association, "Transplant Insurance Studied," *Hospital Week* 19 (23 September 1983): 4.

5. A. M. Enthoven, *Health Plan* (Boston: Addison-Wesley, 1980).

6. W. McClure, "Structure and Incentive Problems in Economic Regulation of Medical Care," *Health and Society/Milbank Memorial Fund Quarterly* 59 (Spring 1981): 107–44.

7. Most economists believe that government would retain an important role in the health care system, even under procompetitive arrangements. For example, government would still have to fund some research and development activities, which are classically undersupported by the private sector in a competitive marketplace. In addition, some economists believe that government regulation (antitrust regulation) would be necessary to prevent collusion among providers of care and to make certain that competing health care plans provided consumers full and fair information on covered benefits and their costs.

8. N. Daniels, "Equity of Access to Health Care: Some Conceptual and Ethical Issues," *Health and Society/Milbank Memorial Fund Quarterly* 60 (Winter 1982): 51–81.

9. L. D. Brown, "Competition and Health Cost Containment: Cautions and Conjectures," *Health and Society/Milbank Memorial Fund Quarterly* 59 (Spring 1981): 145–89.

10. D. Blumenthal, P. Feldman, and R. Zeckhauser, "Misuse of Technology: A Sympton, Not the Disease," in *Critical Issues in Medical Technology*, ed. B. McNeil and E. Cravalho, pp. 163–74 (Boston: Auburn House, 1982).

11. U.S. Congress, Office of Technology Assessment, *Case Study #9, the Artificial Heart*, p. 13.

12. In choosing whether to *continue* research and development projects, the important consideration is the return on marginal dollars, not whether the project will ultimately pay back its total investment in research and development. Consider, for example, a project that has already cost $100 million and will pay back $11 million if a final $10 million is invested in research and development. That final $10 million should be invested; it will reduce the total loss on the project by $1 million.

13. Say we are considering a research and development investment that would cost $1 million. At its conclusion, we expect a product whose marketing is equally likely to result in net benefits of −$30 million, −$10 million, or $10 million. The optimal strategy is to make the research and development investment and bring the project to market only if it will yield $10 million. That strategy has an expected payoff of (⅓) $10 million − $1 million = $2.33 million. Note that it is worthwhile to proceed with the research and development only because one has the opportunity to decide later whether to bring the product to market.

14. T. C. Schelling examines the closely related problem of managing one's own future behavior. He describes a variety of mechanisms that we employ to keep ourselves from making unwise decisions in the future: "Many of us have little tricks we play on ourselves to make us do things we ought to do or to keep us from the things we have foresworn. We place the alarm clock across the room so we cannot turn if off without getting out of bed. We put things out of sight or out of reach for the moment of temptation. We surrender authority to a trustworthy friend who will police our calories or our cigarettes. People who are chronically late set their watches ahead in hopes of fooling themselves. I heard of a corporate dining room where lunch orders are telephoned in at 9:30; no food is served except what was ordered at that time, not long after breakfast, when food was least tempting and resolve at its highest. A grimmer example is people who have their jaws wired shut" ("The Intimate Contest for Self Command," *The Public Interest* 60 [Summer 1980]: 94–118).

15. H. M. Sapolsky, "Here Comes the Artificial Heart," *The Sciences* (December 1978): 25–27.

16. M. C. Weinstein, "Cost-effective Priorities for Cancer Prevention," *Science* 221 (1 July 1983): 17–23.

17. R. R. Nelson, "Government Support of Technical Progress: Lessons from History," *Journal of Policy Analysis and Management* 2 (1983): 499–514.

18. M. C. Weinstein, "Economic Assessments of Medical Practices and Technologies," *Medical Decision-making* 1 (1981): 309–30.

19. U.S. Congress, Office of Technology Assessment, *The Implications of Cost-effectiveness Analysis of Medical Technology* (Washington, D.C.: Government Printing Office, 1980).

20. U.S. Congress, Office of Technology Assessment, *Case Study #9, the Artificial Heart.*

21. B. A. Weisbrod, *The Economics of Medical Research* (Washington, D.C.: American Enterprise Institute, 1983).

22. R. J. Zeckhauser and D. Shepard, "Where Now for Saving Lives?" *Law and Contemporary Problems* (Fall 1976) 40: 5–45.

23. C. Macek, "Cyclosporine's Acceptance Heralds New Era in Immunopharmacology," *JAMA* 250 (22/29 July 1983): 449–55.

24. Evans, draft of testimony.

25. U.S. Congress, Office of Technology Assessment, *Implications of Cost-effectiveness Analysis*, p. 3.

26. Weinstein, "Economic Assessments of Medical Practices and Technologies," p. 311.

27. U.S. Congress, Office of Technology Assessment, *Case Study #9, the Artificial Heart,* p. 34.

28. S. Carrell, "Costs Mark Debate on Artificial Heart," *American Medical News* 1 (28 January 1983): 40–41.

29. We are arguing that the potential recipients of the artificial heart form a heterogenous population in which different subgroups can expect different benefits and costs from the implantation of the artificial heart. Moreover, as the project scale expands, groups with lower expected benefits and higher expected costs will be recruited into the pool of recipients.

The Machine as Means and End: The Clinical Introduction of the Artificial Heart

STANLEY J. REISER

INTRODUCTION

Living on the brink of the Scientific Revolution, English physician and anatomist William Harvey wrote: "Nature herself is to be addressed; the paths she shows us are to be boldly trodden; for thus, and whilst we consult our proper senses . . . shall we penetrate at length into the heart of her mystery."[1] These words, written at the beginning of the seventeenth century, reach the core of the era's methods and purposes. Turning away from the authority of knowledge that was inscribed in the books of revered scholars of the Classical Age, the new scientists, like Harvey, insisted that but one authority, Nature, could be recognized and be boldly interrogated and perceived directly through the human senses. These investigators believed that methodical scientific inquiry eventually would yield her secrets and permit humans, gradually, to dominate her.

The path to be followed in this journey was a path free of considerations based on aim, meaning, values. Objective scientific technique was to pave the route of discovery. Theoretical disputation and strongly held belief was to give way to facts—objective facts derived from a method that involved the breaking down or analysis of complex parts into their components and developed procedures of testing that controlled all but those few variables that were the focus of study. Subjectivity was to be tolerated only in one parameter—the formulation of hypotheses. From then on methodological rigor took over. It is critical to understand that this search for knowledge depended on a universe free of concern about values and of discussion about the nature of being, because such concerns would undermine the capability of the scientist to judge facts unbiased by personal feeling.

By the twentieth century, the engine of scientific progress moved to high gear and was beginning to produce dramatic changes in the knowledge and therapeutic capacity of medicine. Experimental activities became commonplace in laboratories and hospitals. An article in the journal *Modern Hospital*, published in 1926, proclaimed that "every hospital, be it large or small, can make its contribution to the sum total of human knowledge. . . . The hospital is a depository of human problems. Each patient that passes the admission desk comes into the hospital as a living question mark . . . [setting in motion a] quest for the truth behind [it]."[2]

How extraordinarily difficult it has been for this generation of investigators to reintroduce into discussions about the search for knowledge and truth the matter of values. The ethics revolution of the 1960s focused public attention on values related to every aspect of the medical-scientific enterprise, from the methods of testing hypotheses to the social implications of the discoveries generated by proofs. The threat this seemed to pose to the procedural objectivity of the scientific process has been for many the most disturbing aspect of modern ethical discourse about medical science. It has seemed to some that the three-century effort to purge value-related matters from scientific investigation is basically under attack.

Yet, as many now appreciate, a balancing of scientific purpose and human purpose is necessary, just, and overdue. The dilemma is to bring human values and scientific methods into a relationship that damages the vital structure of neither. The artificial heart is an innovation that provides an important test of our ability to create such a balance.

FROM RESEARCH TO THERAPY

An aspect of this general problem, which the artificial heart brings into clear focus, is the matter of where the boundaries are drawn between laboratory and human experimentation on one side and human experimentation and therapeutic use on the other.

From Animal and Laboratory Experiments to Human Experiments

The matter of when it is appropriate to test an innovation on a human being was a central issue in the decision to place the artificial heart into Barney Clark. The documents I have received about this decision from the University of Utah give me a glimpse into the deliberations concerning it, but only a glimpse. Thus, my remarks on this and other specific aspects of the use here of the artificial heart must be general.

In crossing the border between laboratory and human experimentation, a critical judgment is whether a therapeutic benefit for the patient will result, a benefit that overrides the risks of the action. The acquisition of knowledge should be a derivative of this attempt to benefit. The tangible demonstration of benefit is a crucial yardstick against which to measure the justifications for taking this leap and is an important means of limiting premature human tests.

The decision to proceed from animal to human subjects has, since the mid-1960s, focused primarily on preserving the autonomy of the subject. The development of an elaborate procedural examination of consent forms by institutional review boards and the care given to provide subjects with a full view of experimental benefits and risks are reflections of this. Subjects, we now assert, have an absolute right to knowledge and refusal to participate: experimenters have an absolute obligation to disclose what they know and surmise. However, the patient's consent, by itself, is not an adequate warrant for proceeding ahead with an experiment. The consent procedure is set up as a protection; it is not a mechanism meant to bear the total weight of decision. There are some experiments that should not be done whether or not consent has been given by the subject. Investigators themselves are responsible for assuring that experiments are not conducted in which subjects suffer great harm and receive no benefit and are treated basically as a means.

From Human Research to Human Therapy

Difficulty in deciding on when to allow a human trial is matched by the dilemma of deciding if an experimental technique is ready to be used outside of the investigational setting and become part of regular therapeutics. This decision is complicated not only by the scientific and technological aspects of innovations but also by the rise in the number of institutions and decision makers involved with the use of innovation and their particular concerns about it. Industrial companies that generate technologies; hospitals that purchase and organize technologies; clinicians and patients who form relationships to apply technologies; private insurance companies, government agencies, and corporate health plans that distribute funds to pay for technologies; and professional societies concerned about medical actions—all are vitally involved in assuring the rational and just use of technology.

To decide when an innovation is ready for practice is to address the needs of these many constituencies. We thus must be concerned not only with the variables that have traditionally commanded our attention (i.e., physical safety and efficacy) but also with moral, legal, monetary, and social policy considerations. Ethical analyses, cost-effectiveness analyses, determining the capabilities of practitioners and medical institutions outside of the ideal conditions of the experimental setting to properly apply the innovations—such issues must be considered in depth. Contemporary evaluation of technology requires a far broader view of readiness and a more extensive series of analyses to test it than we had in the past. Experimental settings should now be expected to provide this knowledge, if they are to truly help us to use wisely and humanely the technology being created there.

Compounding the problem of the complexity of the modern evaluation process is the urgency of time. Investors, patients, and health care providers all seek to have new innovations applied without delay. Accordingly, there is a pressing need to develop methodologies and institutional arrangements, far more sophisticated than we currently have, in order to evaluate expeditiously the technologies being created. We also use better systems to follow their effects once in practice, so that we can gauge unanticipated, long-range consequences. With such a means of evaluation in place, we can better consider how fast to bring a technology along. Lacking adequate tools of analysis and decision, systems often slow the pace of innovation today by a resort to procedural devices such as certificate-of-need regulations. Such slow-down tactics usually reflect an ambivalence over the consequences of using the innovation. This ambivalence should be addressed by developing the capability to clearly state what the consequences are and to define a strategy of dealing with them. The absence of a process to help decide how to insert new technologies into the system and to take out the older ones they replace greatly encumbers us. Failure to address this issue leads inexorably to the premature introduction into practice of inadequately evaluated technology, whose test of value is basically conducted in uncontrolled clinical settings.

THERAPY AND PROFIT

This leads me to a second general issue raised by the application of the artificial heart: the relationship between the therapeutic good of the subject and the financial good of the investigators. There has long been an uneasiness about the possibility of a conflict of interest when a physician has a particular financial involvement with a remedy being prescribed. For example, the 1957 Principles of Ethics of the American Medical Association is concerned about this conflict, but indicates physicians can supply such treatments provided they are in the best interests of the patient.

This matter is serious, because it goes to the heart of the value that is the foundation of the association between the patient-subject and physician-investigator—trust. Beneath complex relationships such as those involving high-risk experimental therapeutics, when all is said and done the patient-subject must believe that the motives of the physician-investigators stem from goals that transcend their own gain and that they are keeping steadfastly before them the welfare of the patient. The concept of profession in medicine involves a view that service to patients comes before gain to self. Gain is permissible as long as it is derived only from meeting a true non-self-interested need. This motive of service is one of the key features that distinguishes professions from businesses and should be extended to encompass the search for knowledge.

At the University of Utah, the involvement of key staff with commercial interests tied to the success of the artificial heart, as well as the institution itself, introduces questions of self-gain into this delicate balance. It requires those involved to demonstrate in a continuing fashion that this association is in the best interests of patients or at least that it produces no harm.

THE DESTINY OF THE MACHINES WE BUILD

To the question of how to deal with the ownership of our technologic means must be added the problem of living with them. There is a widespread view abroad that machines are simply things to be manipulated by human agents. Unskillful, mean-spirited, self-serving people, so the view goes, will direct machines to socially undesirable ends. Those with higher motives and purer purposes will make machines into agents of social benefit. This view is flawed. The machines we build are highly directive. For we build into them not only mechanical or electronic powers but our own aspirations. They have powerful symbolic meanings for us as well. Thus, as so often happens, once we gain the capability to act through an instrument made for significant action, the machine takes on a life of its own. The machine demands attention: to improve it, to discuss it, to use it, no matter what. Means and ends come together in the question, Can it work? Overriding the objective to define the effects of its use is the fact that it can be used. Like humans, once created, machines seem to acquire a right to survive, to exist, to try to make their mark. Thus machines can be addictive and compelling.

Machines also can become key agents of a view developed through the Scientific Revolution that nature should be mastered, not lived with. What greater act of domination could we as humans devise than to substitute a machine for the most conspicuous agent of life, the heart? How, once we knew how to do it, could we resist the attempt? The artificial heart, apart from its capabilities, has become for our society the foremost symbol of the ambivalence we carry toward medical technology. The artificial heart is at once a metaphor of concern about unduly sustaining an aging population, the cost of medical care, plunging into technologic creation without adequate thought to consequences, and of an accumulation of means as an end in itself. It stands also as a metaphor of exhilaration about the wonders of our science and technology.

To the credit of the University of Utah, the question of using the artificial heart underwent considerable scrutiny, aided by a historically fortuitous circumstance, the presence of an institutional review board, a creation of the ethics revolution of the 1960s. There is little question that the introduction of ethics into medical discourse has served to meliorate, but not subdue, the impulse to apply what we know when we know it before we have fully evaluated consequences. "Technical sweetness" was the phrase physicist Robert Oppenheimer used to describe this phenomenon. Dr. William De-Vries during a discussion at this meeting expressed the matter this way: "Technology goes on—unless there are unbearable side effects." Technology represents the triumph of the production of a means—the capacity to build a bridge, design an airplane, construct a heart. A technologically dominated health care system works undaunted to produce ever more effective means. But to what ends? The difficulties are most acute in such a situation when technology and the various disciplines that study human values and goals are not adequately connected. We then create a crucial imbalance of a continually improving technologic means pursuing imprecisely defined ends.

Some believe that technology itself will solve the problems technology creates; however, history clearly shows this "technologic fix" approach is generally wrong. Technology raises issues of use that can be resolved in some dimension by new technologic breakthroughs. But because of the complex effects of technology, it usually requires other disciplinary advances and analyses to deal with them. We cannot today avoid the social, legal, ethical, and economic dimensions of this question.

The Scientific Revolution sought to make science value free. The ethics revolution has sought to reintroduce values into the doing of science and to demonstrate the complementarity of the humanities and sciences and the necessity for their interactive coexistence. The ideal of a value-free science and a compelling desire to apply rapidly what we can produce make for a powerful combination in a modern world in which the capacity to produce innovations may outstrip our capability to wisely integrate them into the fabric of personal life and societal objectives. The creating of technologic means simply comes easier to us than the development of rational and humane ends to apply them.

It is a difficult circumstance to tolerate that we can create more beneficial medical technology than we have social skills or fiscal capability of providing it to those who are in need of it. Our capacity to produce medical technology will grow and present us with continuing dilemmas, particularly those involving monetary costs, which cannot be met simply by policies directed at creating a more efficient use of health resources. The cost-saving of a policy of efficiency implies a basically static system. What we have, however, is an exceedingly dynamic system, producing technologic goods that are beneficial at an ever increasing rate. Their allocation (and the artificial heart is in this vanguard) will require a far-reaching examination of social and individual values underlying the production and use of medical technology as well as new calculations about the proportion of our nation's wealth we choose to expend on health care.

CONCLUSION

In the first chapter of *De Motu Cordis*, William Harvey wrote:

When I first gave my mind to vivisections, as a means of discovering the motions and uses of the heart, and sought to discover these from actual inspection, and not from the writings of others, I found the task so truly arduous, so full of difficulties, that I was almost tempted to think, with Fracastorius, that the motion of the heart was only to be comprehended by God. For I could neither rightly perceive at first when the systole and when the diastole took place, nor when and where dilation and contraction occurred, by reason of the rapidity of the motion, which in many animals is accomplished in the twinkling of an eye, coming and going like a flash of lightning; so that the systole presented itself to me now from this point, now from that; the diastole the same; and then everything was reversed, the motions occurring, as it seemed, variously and confusedly together. My mind was therefore greatly unsettled, nor did I know what I should myself conclude, nor what to believe from others.[3]

Ultimately Harvey triumphed. Were he to visit us here, he surely would be gratified to learn of the progress we have made since his time toward solving the technical, means-directed problems of heart function that his work so greatly influenced. But he would be startled to find that they have been replaced by social and humanistic ends-directed dilemmas of using these discoveries, which yet leave us moderns, as he himself felt at a crucial stage in his efforts, "greatly unsettled."

NOTES

1. William Harvey, as quoted in George Schwartz and Philip Bishop, eds., *Moments of Discovery: The Development of Modern Science* (New York: Basic Books, 1958), p. 575.

2. Alphonse M. Schwitalla, "The Real Meaning of Research and Why It Should Be Encouraged," in *Ethics in Medicine: Historical Perspectives and Contemporary Concerns*, ed. Stanley Joel Reiser, Arthur J. Dyck, and William J. Curren, p. 264 (Cambridge: MIT Press, 1977).

3. Harvey, as quoted in Schwartz and Bishop, *Moments of Discovery*, p. 575.

Replacing Organs and Replacing Genes

C. THOMAS CASKEY

I have been asked by the conference organizers to discuss medical genetics, an area of medicine that is rapidly advancing and is facing many issues that are similar to those posed by others at this conference on the artificial heart. Geneticists share the frustrations of the cardiac team in our patient care responsibilities. Frequently the complications of genetic disease are beyond help by present treatment modalities. We also share an excitement that new technologies promise hope for presently hopeless patients.[1] The approaches for treatment of heritable diseases by organ and gene replacement differ technically from artificial heart implantation, but they raise many of the same fundamental ethical and medical questions. We wish the therapy to do no harm, to benefit patients, to be highly efficient, and to be cost-effective. Organ replacement and artificial cardiac implantation differ markedly from gene replacement in one major consideration—the potential effects on future generations. It is this last concern that has received the major publicity in articles about genetic engineering.

I would like to review for you some of the different medical and scientific issues that are faced in the medical genetics field. Perhaps this detour from the main consideration—the artificial heart—will help us to put in perspective the commonality of our hopes and fears and frustrations when introducing high-tech medical innovations with potentially far-reaching consequences. I must acknowledge at the outset, however, that we are not as far along in our goals of repairing, replacing, and regulating defective genes as you have progressed in replacing the heart. But we are gaining momentum and making rapid progress.

Gene replacement for heritable disease will not be a single technique, as perhaps cardiac implantation may be. Man has one hundred to two hundred thousand genes encoded in ten trillion base pairs of genetic material, the DNA (deoxyribonucleic acid) in each cell nucleus. We presently recognize about three thousand heritable diseases, but the genetic defect is understood at the molecular level in only several hundred. This number, however, is rapidly increasing as new diagnostic methods become available. Central to these new developments is the area of recombinant DNA technology. Drs. H. Smith and D. Nathans were first to discover a class of enzymes, called restriction endonucleases, that have the ability to cleave the complex DNA molecule at precise sites. These cleavage sites are identical in DNA from bacteria, man, and drosophila. Since the cleavage gives "sticky" ends to the DNA, such fragments from different species can be joined chemically, thus forming new recombinant DNA molecules. Acquiring the ability to form recombinant molecules was rapidly followed by our acquiring the ability to replicate them in microbes. Dr. S. Cohen was first to discover that recombinant DNA molecules inserted into microbial plasmids made possible their replication in large quantity. Thus small amounts of DNA, when inserted into plasmids, permitted cloning and amplification of the recombinant form. Dr. F. Blattner further improved on this cloning technology by the use of bacteriophage cloning methods. These highly efficient methods permit cloning of long sequences, starting with a very small amount of DNA. It has become possible to deposit in a "bank" all of the DNA content of a single individual by storing each segment with a separate identification or "account" number. Drs. F. Sanger and W. Gilbert provided the methods for sequencing this genetic material, or breaking the genetic code of each fragment. These combined technologies of cloning and sequencing have been applied to the analysis of certain hemoglobin diseases, resulting in the successful identification of twenty-six different mutations accounting for the single class of diseases called β-thalassemia (caused by a defect of the β-globin portion of the hemoglobin molecule).

In addition to helping us understand genetic diseases, DNA technology has provided us with a way of increasing the efficiency of production of several pharmaceutical agents. Growth hormone and insulin synthesized by recombinant DNA techniques have been released by the Food and Drug Administration for human use. The diagnosis of heritable defects has represented still another major successful application of this technology. The prenatal diagnosis of the hemoglobinopathies has been greatly simplified by analyzing DNA from amniotic cells after certain restriction endonucleases have fragmented the DNA. This brief review illustrates the dramatic and rapid effect of DNA recombinant technology on heritable disease understanding, diagnosis, and prevention.

One might ask whether efforts at gene replacement therapy are misdirected if the preventive approaches, such as prenatal diagnosis, look so promising. I do not believe we should take this position toward gene therapy, just as I would argue that one cannot take exclusively a preventive approach to cardiac disease. Let me illustrate the problems in implementing prevention of heritable disease by a discussion of autosomal recessive disorders. Sickle-cell disease, β-thalassemia, Tay-Sachs, cystic fibrosis, mucopolysaccharidosis, and gangliosidosis are examples of severe disorders inherited by an autosomal recessive mechanism. For the first three listed, simple, cheap, and reliable methods of identifying carriers are available. These diseases are common to certain ethnic groups: blacks, mediterranean peoples, and Ashkenazi Jews, respectively. Also, each of these three is amenable to prenatal diagnosis. This combination of circumstances provides an optimal opportunity for disease prevention by population screening, counseling of couples at risk, and prenatal diagnosis. These approaches have been sufficiently tested and evaluated, but there are several major drawbacks to the successful implementation of these preventive programs: patient and physician education; patient and physician acceptance; and patient acceptance of the reproductive alternatives of adoption, artificial insemination by donor, and prenatal diagnosis followed by selective abortion of defective fetuses. Although the approach has proved extremely effective in the prevention of Tay-Sachs disease, affected children continue to be born to parents who have not participated in the prevention efforts.

There remains a need for developing treatment modalities for these "preventable" as well as for many other recessive diseases for which no carrier detection method exists, the gene frequency is very low, or prenatal diagnosis is not available. We will continue to identify couples with genetic risk by diagnosis of their "index case" offspring. We are faced with additional reasons for failure of prevention approaches in the circumstances in which the disease occurs by new mutation. This would include diseases such as Duchenne type muscular dystrophy and Lesch-Nyhan syndrome, both X-linked recessive disorders. Since a large number of these cases (70–90 percent) represent a new mutational event rather than inheritance of an abnormal gene, no opportunity for the above preventive approaches exists. I, therefore, conclude that it is impractical to use prevention of heritable disease as the sole or even major means of disease control. The recombinant DNA technology area offers an alternative gene replacement therapy.

My laboratory has devoted considerable effort toward this objective for the Lesch-Nyhan syndrome.[2] This disorder is inherited as an

X-linked recessive disease and is characterized by mental retardation, severe uncontrolled movements, and self-destructive behavior. We have successfully applied molecular techniques toward isolation of the normal gene from human DNA that is allelic to the defective Lesch-Nyhan gene. This has been done both from messenger RNA and nuclear DNA. The normal base sequence, as well as the molecular defect in twelve different families with the disease, is now known. These developments have led to improved carrier detection methods for females in 60 percent of these families.

Our recent efforts have been directed toward gene replacement. I would like to briefly report these results. "Mini-genes" are now available that contain both regulatory elements and gene-coding sequences. These recombinant molecules have been used successfully to transfer the normal gene into defective Lesch-Nyhan cells in culture. Transfer is successful by calcium precipitation or microinjection methods. More recently, construction of the mini-gene into defective retrovirus virions has succeeded. Although this success is quite exciting, we should examine our original objectives in gene replacement therapy.

Can harm be done by this approach? Our studies indicate that the mini-genes take up residence in the replacement cell by "illegitimate" recombination. Thus, new genes are inserted randomly and do not vector to the resident defective gene location. This poses the problem of introducing new mutations elsewhere in the DNA; in fact, such an untoward effect has been demonstrated in separate studies in mice. It is not known what the practical risk of this event will be to a patient. Additional studies in mice must be carried out before introducing replacement genes in man. Can harm be done to future generations? The techniques now under consideration for man are directed toward patient not embryo treatment. There is clear evidence that introduction of new genes into mouse embryos can be detected in the adult mouse and its progeny. No evidence exists that similar entry of new genes into gonadal tissues occurs when adult animals are treated. The issue deserves further study because experience is limited.

Can the patient benefit from the therapy? This is a difficult question for heritable diseases. For cardiac failure, replacement of the pump is anticipated to provide clinical improvement. Although gene defects exist in all cells of the patient, the disease is usually manifested in one or several target tissues. In the case of Lesch-Nyhan disease, it is the central nervous system and kidney. In the case of phenylketonuria, it is the liver and central nervous system. In the case of sickle-cell disease, it is the blood cells in the bone marrow. These examples serve to illustrate the problem of achieving clinical improvement. Delivery of the gene to the improper tissue may not only not achieve patient improvement but could potentially complicate the disorder. Each disease will differ in this regard. Organ replacement by transplantation has provided a simple solution for some genetic diseases. Successful treatment of the renal heritable diseases of Fabry's and polycystic kidney disease has been achieved by renal transplantation, alpha₁-antitrypsin deficiency by liver transplantation, and immune deficiency disease by marrow transplantation. These approaches suffer from the problems associated with immune rejection, just as do cardiac transplants. No simple single approach to correction exists presently for heritable diseases, either by gene or organ replacement.

Can the replacement gene be delivered with high efficiency? Cells cultured from the patient can be used as recipients of new genes and then delivered in a variety of ways. The efficiency of each method differs. Gene transfer by calcium precipitation is practical in cultured cells but would appear impractical for human use because of its low efficiency. Gene transfer by microinjection is unable to transfer genes to large numbers of cells in a short time. It is, however, highly efficient for the injected cell. Recently, defective retroviruses have been used for transfer of the Lesch-Nyhan gene into cultured cells. It is highly efficient (one virus equals one gene transfection) and appears most promising at this time. In none of the approaches above have we solved the problems of cell specificity for gene transfer. The methods for precise delivery to brain, liver, or bone marrow cells are unresolved. The work has progressed to successful transfer of genes into mouse embryos and blood-forming cells of adult mice.

I would like to briefly review the progress on transfer of genes to mouse embryos. R. Brinster and R. Palmiter have developed microinjection techniques that are successful in 25 percent of embryos injected. The adult animals derived from these studies can be found to have the transgene in all body tissues, including gonadal tissues. The newly acquired gene sequence is transmitted to progeny as a mendelian unit. Thus, in one step—microinjection—new genes are acquired by the mouse. Study of these animals indicates that the foreign genes have variable expression in different tissues and lack normal control. Furthermore, it has been demonstrated that newly acquired genes have recombined with other functional genes, leading to new mutations in the mouse. Thus, the data in this experimental system are not sufficiently promising to seriously consider embryo injection for man. There are several other practical issues that further reduce the potential usefulness of this procedure for man. For autosomal or X-linked recessive disease, the odds favor normality (3 : 4). The affected embryo occurs at a frequency of 1 : 4. Thus, introduction of foreign genes into embryos at risk but not diagnosed would lead to transgene introduction to many normal individuals. Microdiagnostic methods to distinguish the affected from unaffected would further complicate the process. Thus, in my opinion, both on practical and ethical considerations, the introduction of genes into human embryos is premature.

The potential of gene transfer in therapy of heritable diseases is rapidly developing. We have succeeded in transferring normal human genes into cells in culture and into mice. We have identified the predominant mechanism of gene integration and determined the level of expression. These results are encouraging. In some cases, the severity of disease will justify application of these new approaches to man. Such studies will need to be carefully designed to provide an understanding of the measurements of intermediate events leading to successful therapy. But knowledge is presently inadequate to predict successful cure of disease by these methods. Despite these reservations, it is clear that a number of investigative groups have the vision, objective, and technical capacity to develop this new therapeutic method.

The work of the medical geneticist, like the work of the implant surgeon, will undoubtedly be carried out in the glare of the public limelight. This is because of its creative appeal and also because it raises the specter of tinkering with Nature in heretofore unthinkable ways. That is the price we must be willing to pay for medical progress, and it is only proper that the public be a partner with us in our ventures into the unknown.

NOTES

1. C. T. Caskey and R. L. White, eds., *Banbury Report 14: Recombinant DNA Applications to Human Disease* (Cold Spring Harbor, N.Y.: Cold Spring Harbor Laboratory, 1983), pp. 81–89.

2. C. T. Caskey, T. P. Yang, P. I. Patel, J. T. Stout, and A. C. Chinault, "The Characterization and Correction of Lesch-Nyhan gene defects by Recombinant DNA techniques," in *Advances in Gene Technology: Human Genetic Disorders, Proceedings of the 16th Miami Winter Symposium*, ed. Fazal Ahmad, Sandra Black, Julius Schultz, Walter A. Scott, and William J. Whelan, International Council of Scientific Unions (ICSU) Short Reports, vol. 1 (Miami: ICSU Press, 1984).

Summary of Discussion on Economic, Historical, and Scientific Issues

JOANN ELLISON RODGERS

OVERVIEW AND BACKGROUND

In describing one speaker's presentation as an "intellectual pep-talk," Cornell's Eric Cassell unwittingly supplied a useful, if not literal, framework in which the conference's final session can be placed. In the formal presentations and the informal discussion that followed, the message was on balance upbeat. Each speaker in his or her way reaffirmed the view that people of intellect and thoughtfulness can and should harness medical technology, scientific process, and ethical values to serve the needs of individuals and society. If no one on the Utah heart team or the University of Utah Institutional Review Board for Research with Human Subjects (IRB) came away from the session with a no-fault game plan or a directed victory, most at least seemed eager to suit up for the second half.

In the context of the conference's design (to offer debate rather than instruction), this final session was not only predictable but also somewhat cathartic. The previous day's discussions had focused tightly on the Barney Clark case, triggering inevitable tensions and disagreements but proscribing the sense of relief or accomplishment that would have come with what Albert Jonsen referred to as "closure or resolution." Added to the tension was the almost palpable concern among members of the heart team, the IRB, and makers of the Jarvik-7 heart over growing social criticism of their entire program.

While closure and resolution remained elusive at the end, the final day's discussion was given over to broader perspectives, which provided an emotional buffer, drained off tension, and left conferees with an overall positive feeling about the experience. Specifically, the last conference session introduced the economics of emerging technology, the historical roots of our commitment to the "technological fix," and the development of the science of gene replacement as both analog for the *therapia exotica* of the artificial heart and paradigm for public policy considerations.

ECONOMIC ISSUES IN DEVELOPING TECHNOLOGIES

David Blumenthal, a physician with broad experience in public policy and economics, explored the economic issues that characterize rapidly emerging medical technologies. Among other things, the artificial heart *is* an economic issue. An overriding concern is when to apply cost-benefit analysis as a policy-making tool: During research and development? If so, when? Or must it be postponed until a device or procedure such as the artificial heart develops sufficiently to create market demand? His point of departure was not classical or marketplace economics but a broader definition of economics that pays attention to shifting social and human values and the concept of getting our money's worth even if the expenditure is huge or uncertain. The artificial heart program, he noted, is especially pertinent to this view of economics because it pulls certain economic decisions into an extraordinarily symbolic and metaphorical debate over human values and the worth of human life.

As a society, Blumenthal noted, we've paid "heavily" to preserve the myth that life is worth any cost. And developing a pro–artificial heart policy, with all the attendant demands for equitable distribution and pay schemes, makes "the price of preserving that myth . . . exorbitant." Indeed, he said, "the artificial heart . . . may prove to be the first instance in which . . . the price of preserving the myth that life is priceless may prove too high."

The science and art of economics, he added, can contribute to the debate and help health policymakers make tough choices among tough alternatives by clarifying the organization and effects of financing our health care system. Economists are interested in using resources efficiently, he said, not just in reducing costs. There is recognition of the reality of scarcity, not penury. Economics, he added, will never provide unequivocal numerical decisions about whether to proceed and use the artificial heart, but it does have valuable insights to offer in thinking about whether and how to proceed with the development of the artificial heart and how to use it if and when it becomes available. Its value is to help illuminate uncertainties and hidden problems. To demonstrate his points about economics, Blumenthal first reviewed guesstimates of dollar costs associated with the artificial heart program, among them John Bunker's estimate of $28,000 per implant and the potential number of candidates, placed at from 16,000 to 66,000 a year in the under–sixty-five population of cardiovascular disease victims.

Drawing again on Bunker's data, Blumenthal's cost-benefit analysis (with co-author Richard Zeckhauser) suggested that at $28,000 per device and implant operation and a $2,000 per year maintenance cost for five years, the annual dollar cost of a comprehensive artificial heart program in the United States would be $1.1 billion for 33,600 patients. That price would purchase approximately one to four years of additional life for selected individuals, but overall would increase the life expectancy of the average twenty-five–year–old American by only seven to thirty-five days. The artificial heart could be an exception to the unwritten rule that new technologies that work tend to spread rapidly. But if it isn't, the implications in terms of cost could be staggering. A small federal research budget may balloon into billions of dollars in later costs, as was (and is) the case with the kidney dialysis and transplant program. In sum, he said, because of its "symbolic value, its life-giving potential, and its daunting potential costs, the artificial heart epitomizes the trade-offs inherent in extending life through extraordinary means."

Next Blumenthal discussed the influence of currently powerful economists on the financial structure of our health care system. This cadre of individuals would reform the system by fostering free market competition in the health care sector, competition they believe will best determine the value and distribution of devices and services. With respect to the artificial heart, this approach would, if it worked, find consumers who wanted the option of an implant to purchase health plans that would cover one. And if the price proved unacceptable, consumer interest would fall. In order for a health plan to remain competitive and viable, it would discontinue such coverage, and the artificial heart program would "wither."

The point to remember, he said, is that the organization of the health care system, whether a competitive model or some other, has a lot to say about the development of any new health care technology and that solving problems in the artificial heart program may, at least in part, depend on solving structural problems within the health care system. He also warned that the artificial heart should not be used as an argument for or against a national health insurance program. The artificial heart should be judged, from an economics viewpoint, on its own merits or lack of them, and not used as a flying wedge for regulatory initiatives.

Subsequently, Blumenthal considered the difficulties of comparing alternatives when the outcome of using or not using a particular technology is life or death. Equally difficult is the anticipation of spin-offs from and improvements in the artificial heart research and development project that could be used to offset both dollar and social costs of the project. Perhaps, Blumenthal concluded, if the health care system were better and properly organized in the first place, economic scenarios could be analyzed and tested with more confidence and accuracy: "If our system embodied more appropriate financial incentives concerning the use of health care technologies, we could be far more relaxed and permissive in our treatment of research and development projects."

But clearly we do not have this situation. What do we do? Leave the money spigot open because we fear cutting off some valuable project prematurely? Set strict budget priorities? Blumenthal said he favors the latter solution, but only, he emphasized, when a project is in the applied stage should it be subjected to strict priority screening. Moreover, cost-benefit analysis should never be the only criterion for survival. Opportunity costs of the artificial heart, the benefits that might have been realized from alternative uses of investment resources, must also be factored in, and these may be extremely difficult to calculate. Blumenthal gave the following illustration: Some proponents of the artificial heart note that our health care system might provide an implant for all candidates for the price of a single nuclear-powered aircraft carrier. The economic fallacy here is the assumption that the resources used to develop the artificial heart would be drawn from the military budget. In reality, the project is more likely to drain limited dollars from research and programs that would do far more toward preventing disease and preserving health in the population. Not recognizing this point could lead to a serious underestimate of opportunity costs. It is almost certain, Blumenthal said, that the artificial heart will fall into the category of devices that extend life but at a significant cost, forcing it to be one of a number of projects competing for limited dollars.

In the audience discussion that followed, Alexander Capron pointed out that the "myth" of life's infinite preservation costs doesn't exact any cost in our ethical system until the health care system can actually do something. There was no ethical impetus for early-stage development of the artificial heart or liver transplantation. No one considered it sinful or immoral that such therapies were unavailable. Only when a useful therapy comes along and carries a huge price tag do we face the ethical challenge inherent in the myth. "As long as liver transplantation was still rare and highly experimental, there was little sense that the failure to provide one was [ethically] wrong," Capron noted. But now, as it has turned the corner to therapy, "we have a public circus," and people are asking how anyone can refuse to provide liver transplants.

Blumenthal replied by suggesting that economic and ethical "monitoring" be employed whenever a new technology emerges and preferably at the earliest stages. He would make this recommendation even though we would be at risk of prematurely giving up a valuable innovation in order to avoid certain ethical and dollar costs. Robert Jarvik argued that valid cost-benefit analysis is impossible until the artificial heart program gets beyond the first few cases, because the earliest patients are always the least likely to survive or benefit over a long period. Early analysis should be confined, he said, to aiding decisions about *how* to proceed, not *whether* to proceed.

Blumenthal, however, considered that approach a cop-out. There are ways, imperfect though they are, of coping with and incorporating uncertainties about patient selection into cost-benefit formulas. If we just opt out of trying, because of the difficulties and the risks of error, we will be overwhelmed by costs we have never even tried to anticipate. At present, he said, "We are contorting ourselves to find ways of analyzing the costs of research and development because we are fearful of what will happen economically if a technology becomes available." He agreed that "ideally, perhaps the consumer should be the throttle" on the money engine, but he added that there is "no incentive" in our health care system for this approach. The consumer won't take social costs into account because under our insurance reimbursement system, he is not made to bear any personal costs. Blumenthal insisted that although our system of funding technological progress will never be perfect, "it can do better," and, he added, "historically, [funding] has been done pretty well."

WHAT CAN WE LEARN FROM THE PAST?

Shifting gears to a historical perspective, physician and medical historian Stanley J. Reiser traced the roots of the artificial heart debate to a fundamental, developmental dichotomy in science. When William Harvey first made the function of the heart the object of hands-on, direct investigation, his achievements were stunning, in great part because his approach signaled and encouraged the Scientific Revolution. His empiricism, his passion for objective facts, stood in stark contrast to the Classical Age of subjectivity in science from which he emerged in the seventeenth century. Experimentation became de rigueur and subjectivity—philosophical consideration—was overthrown as a major impetus to scientific thought and achievement.

"Turning away from the authority of knowledge that was inscribed in the books of revered scholars of the Classical Age," Reiser said, "the new scientists, like Harvey, insisted that but one authority, Nature, could be recognized and be boldly interrogated and perceived directly through the human senses." Then he added that the true path of science became a path free of such considerations as motive, meaning, and value. Such considerations were considered strangling, incompatible with truth finding.

By the twentieth century, the revolution was mature. Science had shifted from a personally satisfying to an other-directed, transcendent activity. Thus, it should come as no surprise to anyone involved in the artificial heart debate that practitioners of science now find it difficult to reintroduce the idea of personal values and ethics into the proceedings. Science as we have known it for three hundred years, Reiser explained, is now thought by some of its practitioners to be threatened by a virtual bombardment from the bioethics community. The task today, he suggested, is to bring both ethics and the traditional scientific method together without damaging either, since both have advantages and contributions to make.

In a far-ranging and entertaining presentation, Reiser concluded that the artificial heart is a major test of our ability as a society to accomplish that task, to determine boundaries, to set patient selection criteria that are both humane and scientifically sound, to permit free scientific choice and pursuit of profit while still paying attention in depth to legal, moral, economic, ethical, and social needs. He dealt also with the issue of trust and the changing role of the scientist-entrepreneur. Patients, he said, hold the view that personal gain for a scientist is fine as long as the gain emerges from service to them, not from a purely business arrangement. Any other approach injects a potential conflict of interest for the medical scientist that patients perceive as compromising their own interests. Reiser then turned to an examination of the common view that machines are simply things to be manipulated by people and if the people doing the manipulating are pure and unselfish, the machines' use will be likewise. Such a view, according to Reiser, is dangerously flawed, and it was at this point that his presentation segued from a comfortable base of history and contemporary observation to a controversial, exciting, and challenging conclusion.

Reiser argued that the machines we build are "highly directive," for we build them to reflect our own, very human, aspirations; that they have symbolic meaning; that a look at our machines tells us much about our societal values and where we are going, as well as where we came from. He had merged the technological fix with social theory and uncovered both in a powerful new form of cybernetics and a new challenge for the subjective-objective dilemma faced by modern scientists.

"Once we gain the capability to act through an instrument, . . . the machine takes on a life of its own," he said. He explained that the machine "demands attention: to improve it, to discuss it, to use it, no matter what." The objective becomes not to define the effects of its use but to prove the fact that it can be used. In that sense, our machines acquire certain inalienable rights no less than their users. Among them is the right to survive. Reiser added that machines have become "addictive and compelling," agents of a view that "nature should be mastered, not lived with." He presented the dilemma: "What greater act of domination could we as humans devise than to substitute a machine for the most conspicuous agent of human life, the heart. How, once we knew how to do it, could we resist the attempt?"

One consequence of the attempt is that the artificial heart has become a metaphor for fears about unduly sustaining an aging population, for plunging into fearsome technologies without sufficient thought for the consequences, and for the exhilaration that accompanies the wonders of science and the high-tech fix. In a society that has become medicalized, willing to believe that our scientific experts can and should cure every human frailty and unhappiness, the empirical scientist, including those who pursue the artificial heart, are at ease and invested with high status. "Technology goes on," he quoted a member of the artificial heart team, "unless there are unbearable side effects."

But as Reiser pointed out, history teaches us that the technological fix requires input from social, legal, economic, and ethical caretakers if the fix is to benefit; otherwise, it may control us, instead of the other way around. But to the degree we are willing at all to solve the problems of the artificial heart program, we bear witness to a commitment to merge science and the humanities. The ideal of a value-free science, he concluded, promotes a powerful capability to make machines, but not for using them very wisely for humane and rational ends. William Harvey, he noted, would be gratified to· learn of our progress in understanding the mechanics of heart disease, a journey his work greatly influenced, but he would be startled to find so much concern about the use of these discoveries.

It was during the discussion that Reiser's interest in the artificial heart project and the possibilities that project represents for merging science and the humanities came across most forcefully. It represented, he noted, an awesome power and willingness to confront some of the most fearsome symbols of man's vulnerability.

Cassell explored the idea with Reiser that in the rise of science, machines have been seen as a danger, with Frankenstein's monster the quintessential example of how scientific tinkering results in unrestrained humanity. "Is the artificial heart like this?" he asked. Are those who use it seen as untrustworthy, as monsters that would overrun mere mortals? Cassell saw the IRB's apparent mistrust of its own scientists as evidence that the artificial heart is seen that way.

Reiser agreed with Cassell, up to a point, acknowledging that we have a love-hate relationship with our machines. We love them, but we fear them. But, in fact, what we worry about is our own ability to control ourselves. Though we see the enormous benefit in our machines, we fear, and with good reason, the power they give us. But for all of the fears, the scientific method survives and proceeds and evolves to meet changing human values and needs, and its practitioners, he suggested, are still invested with enormous status and leeway.

THE FASCINATION OF FUTURE TECHNOLOGIES

The audience wondered, as C. Thomas Caskey began his presentation on genetic engineering, what relevance his subject had to artificial hearts. But it proved to offer a stunning look at what could be the future concerns of the artificial heart program. The medical geneticist, Caskey explained, like the heart specialist, has long been one of a group of frustrated physicians whose patients are sick or dying and who have no solutions. Again, like the heart specialist, the medical geneticist now has access to technologies (in this case recombinant DNA and hybridomas instead of machines) that offer hope where once there was no hope. Where the artificial heart is a mechanical solution, genetic therapy is a molecular solution. Philosophically, the heart and the genetic domain of the cell nucleus are both, in a way, analogs of the soul. Each of us is concerned about not doing harm, about benefiting patients, and about being efficient, Caskey said, carrying the similarities between cardiac surgeon and medical geneticist further.

Granted there are differences. When an artificial heart fails, the experiment and the therapy for that patient end, along with life. In gene therapy, there is potential for doing greater harm to the patient if it fails and the patient is forced to live with the failure. Worse, the experiment may not end with that patient but be carried to future generations. Finally, the geneticist's target "organ" is an entire physiological system, not a single mechanical unit. The complexities of sorting out which functional gene must be replaced or repaired are mind-boggling compared with building a mechanical pump. The discovery of restriction enzymes and their subsequent use to recombine and clone DNA sequences have offered a simple but powerful tool for unraveling the complicated human genome.

Caskey gave several examples of how new genetic technologies are beginning to be applied to genetic diseases. Antenatal testing combined with selective abortion have been commonplace approaches to a multitude of rare genetic and chromosomal disorders. Now the common hematogenetic diseases, sickle-cell anemia and the β-thalassemias, are succumbing to fetal diagnosis through restriction enzyme analysis. The normal gene for Lesch-Nyhan disease, a self-mutilating disorder, has been cloned and transferred into cultured cells from these patients, resulting in cellular correction of the enzyme deficiency. There are also on the horizon several viral systems that will be capable of delivering a normal gene to the target cells of patients with a gene defect that causes disabling disease.

Cloned populations of genes responsible for Duchenne type muscular dystrophy and inborn errors of metabolism and enzyme storage diseases are either near at hand or have been achieved. The excitement within the medical genetics community is enormous, just as it is among the artificial heart program participants. But the uncertainties of gene therapy, coupled with the potential to do more harm than good, have provided a brake on the use of these new technologies that Caskey not only accepts but finds reassuring. He did not mean to imply that medical geneticists have given up the dream of gene therapy, but the therapy will almost certainly, in the immediate future, rely on organ transplants from normal individuals to individuals with inherited defects. The successful transplantation of cloned genes to patients with alpha$_1$-antitrypsin deficiency represents such an example. This approach lacks the precision of gene transfers but buys time for the geneticist to study long-term consequences. At the same time, Caskey suggested, the emotional, social, and economic issues raised by rapid advances in genetics have led to wider public discussion and acceptance of approaches to genetic disease once seen as politically impossible, such as genetic screening and selective abortion.

In the discussion that followed Caskey's remarks, Margery Shaw explained that medical genetics is an apt paradigm for the artificial heart program because the former stimulated discussion of public fears about utility at a very early stage in development. Those fears, reflected in scare scenarios in the media, threatened at many stages to cut off funding for genetic research. Only when the prospects for successfully treating children with dread diseases emerged was the public interest calmed and focused.

There was a clear suggestion in this discussion that when defenders of the artificial heart program seek public sympathy for their project as a therapy, rather than a piece of gee-whiz experimental technology, they will find themselves better able to advance their cause with policymakers and research budget directors. The National Institutes of Health recently held an open forum called "Gene Transfer: A Method for Treatment of Heritable Disease." Medical genetics is meeting this challenge, it seems, and so probably can the artificial heart program.

A FINAL WORD

The ultimate utility of the final presentations and discussion was and is debatable in this reporter's opinion. In a group as highly task-oriented as the one gathered by the conference organizers, it was difficult for many to whom I spoke to find a hand- or toe-hold for easing the way out of a frustrating, self-imposed moratorium on the Utah project. At the time of the conference, remember, ten months had passed since University of Utah surgeons performed the world's first artificial heart implant, and prospects for a second were still on hold. Despite the planning that had gone into the selection and treatment of Barney Clark, six months of evaluations, and the apparent success of the Jarvik-7 device itself, most of the ticklish and complicated social problems posed by the Utah project were no closer to solution. "We came to this conference of national experts," said IRB chairman John Bosso, "looking for a guide to smoother roads for the heart team, and we learned that we will still have to muddle through pretty much by ourselves." Nevertheless, in a widespread sentiment voiced most articulately by Ross Woolley, former chairman of the heart subcommittee of the IRB, the mood was positive. He said, "We have learned that no outside experts or consultants can do our job for us. That's all right. We can and will do it ourselves."

The conferees' interest in the exercise offered by the last day's session and the optimism it bred were sufficient to earn it a memorable niche in the proceedings.

Appendixes

Appendix A

SPECIAL CONSENT FOR
ARTIFICIAL HEART DEVICE IMPLANTATION
AND RELATED PROCEDURES

1.1 The undersigned understands that on the basis of various diagnostic procedures, that I have a condition known as [END STAGE CHRONIC CONGESTIVE FAILURE SECONDARY TO IDIOPATHIC CARDIOMYOPATHY]

(describe condition)

which has so seriously impaired the function of my heart that I have been placed in category IV of the New York Heart Association which states:

"Class IV patients have the inability to carry on any physical activity without discomfort. Symptoms of discomfort are present even at rest. With any physical activity, increased discomfort is experienced."

It is the judgment of physicians and others who have evaluated my diagnostic tests that, although no specific life span can be estimated, it is probable that I will die much sooner than most others of my age and that while alive I will continue to be severely restricted due to my failing heart. I further understand that there are no further medical therapies that will arrest the course of this deterioration of my heart. Replacement of my natural heart is the only treatment. While prolongation of life beyond that expected for my condition by use of a mechanical heart has not been proven in humans, nevertheless I am willing to submit to its implantation on an experimental basis in order to determine if it will help people with my condition.

With these considerations in mind, and with the further understanding and recognition of the additional matters contained in this document, I hereby authorize Dr. William C. DeVries, who is referred to hereafter in this special consent as "my physician," and such assistants and associates as he may designate, to implant a mechanical artificial heart in place of my diseased natural heart. Any consideration as to my selection for a heart transplant procedure would be determined by an independent cardiac transplantation team from another medical center. I understand that if I do not meet their criteria for a future heart transplant, I must accept the artificial heart as a final life-sustaining device.

It is most probable that the artificial heart will be a final life-sustaining device for an undefined period.

1.2   I also understand that laboratory and animal testing suggest that implantation of an artificial heart device in some cases may provide sufficient circulatory support to sustain life for a limited but indefinite period. Therefore the artificial heart may function as a temporary life-support system for an indefinite period of time in the hope a donor heart can be secured and my selection made for transplantation. However, I understand that I may not qualify for heart transplantation and no assurances have been made to me regarding my selection for a heart transplantation operation.

2.1   I hereby request and authorize my physician to proceed with the implantation of an experimental total artificial heart device. I <u>recognize that the ventricles</u> (the larger two of the heart's four pumping chambers) <u>from my own natural heart will be removed</u> and a mechanical heart device will be placed within my chest in the space formerly occupied by my own natural heart, and that this mechanical device will require my body to be attached to an air-driving system by two plastic six-foot long air tubes to pump my blood through my mechanical heart and circulate it through my body. I am aware that my life style will be significantly different with an artificial heart. My activity will be <u>severely limited</u> because of the drive lines. The external drive systems will not necessarily require me to be bedridden but at best would allow me to move from room to room, and may allow brief periods of being outside and riding in a car or van if it is capable of carrying the external drive system. I may be able to carry on many life functions in a normal manner (e.g. toilet activity, eating, reading and desk work). It is possible, however, that I may have to remain bedridden due to pain, weakness or other problems.

2.2   I further understand that due to the positioning and nature of the artificial heart if it is installed, that in addition to the surgery necessary for the original installation, additional chest surgeries may be required in the event the device needs to be replaced or repaired which will be explained to me and will be done with a new consent form signed by me for each such procedure and that in all likelihood, general anesthesia with its attendant risks would be necessary in connection with such procedures.

2.3   I also understand that if the artificial heart device is installed that I can anticipate considerable postoperative pain and discomfort similar to or greater than that which would be experienced following the usual type of cardiovascular surgery, and that additional or prolonged discomfort and pain may result in the event of further surgery. I also understand that the use of the artificial heart may necessitate additional instrumentation and studies in order that adequate information may be obtained concerning its functioning, and such instrumentation and studies are expected to consist of or be similar to those involved in cardiac catheterization but may include other procedures, with attendant risks, discomfort and inconvenience. Each of these new procedures will have a consent form which must be signed before they are performed.

3. I recognize that during the course of the operation, unforeseen conditions may necessitate additional or different procedures than those set forth in paragraphs under 2 above. This will be discussed with me, but if at that time I am too sick to be consulted, I further authorize my physicians to perform such procedures as are, in their professional judgment, necessary and desirable. The authority granted under this paragraph 3, shall extend to remedying conditions that are not known at the time the surgery is commenced.

4. I consent to the administration of anesthesia as arranged by my physician with such assistants as may be designated, and to the use of such anesthetics as they may in their judgment deem advisable.

5. I have also been informed of the substantial risks involved in cardiovascular surgery and the administration of general anesthesia, and understand that there are additional risks beyond those normally associated with cardiovascular surgery, as a result of the artificial heart implantation, which may result in serious bodily impairment, or death, such as:

    a. Emboli (release of a thrombus) which may result in stroke, loss of kidneys, liver, bowel, lung or partial impairment of organ or body function.
    b. Malfunction or mechanical failure of the artificial heart device.
    c. Infection of: My blood (sepsis), the driving lines to the artificial heart device or infection of the artificial heart device itself.
    d. Hemorrhage resulting from the action of the artificial heart device upon the vessels, surgery to expose the heart, or other causes.
    e. Damage to the red blood cells (that carry oxygen and carbon dioxide), the platelets (that cause blood to clot) or white blood cells (that act as scavengers against foreign substances and provide for immunization) which might cause a change in my blood immune system or anemia.
    f. Internal hemorrhage due to deficiencies in the blood clotting mechanisms secondary to the artificial heart.
    g. Pneumothorax. Air in the chest cavity which may result in difficulty breathing requiring a separate tube to be placed in my chest.

Because this is a highly experimental procedure there may be other risks which are not foreseeable at this time which may arise and the above items should not be considered as all inclusive only illustrative.

6.1   I further recognize that this procedure is <u>experimental</u>. Similar artificial heart devices have been used only in two living patients in other institutions as a temporary emergency, life-prolonging procedure until a heart transplant could be obtained. The devices used in these patients were not the same as the model which would be used in my case. The artificial heart was removed and a heart transplant performed. Both of these patients died within one week after removal of the artificial heart from complications.

6.2   The University of Utah has had extensive experience with living animals implanted with a similar model of artificial heart as will be used in my case. The present human model has had only limited testing in these animals. However, the device to be used is the most refined and advanced model which is available for use in a human. To date the longest an animal (a calf) has lived with an artificial heart is nine months. Most animals live for about three months in experiments designed to test long-term effects of heart implantation. The poor hygiene of animals makes it very difficult to keep them clean and most die from infections caused by bacteria entering around the drive tubes or other tubes used to monitor the function of the heart. Other common causes of death in these animals are: infected blood obtained from packing houses which is used to transfuse them, insufficient blood volume coming from the heart as the calves grow, and the artificial heart developing mechanical problems. While these complications reflect problems which may be unique to animal experimentation, they also provide additional warnings of risk which should be considered with the potential complications in Section 5.

7.   No representations have been made to me with respect to whether the procedure will be successful, nor the length of time which the artificial heart device will function, nor the level at which it will function. I recognize that if the artificial heart device fails, death or serious injury is the near certain result. I nevertheless accept the risk of substantial and serious harm, including death, in the hope that beneficial effects of the implantation of the artificial heart device can be demonstrated. No guarantees have been made to me concerning the result of the operation or procedure.

8.   I acknowledge that my physician has in a satisfactory manner, explained to me the procedure involved in the implantation of the artificial heart into my body and that all questions that I have asked about the procedure and its attendant risks, including death, the experimental nature of the artificial heart, its expected function, the probable restrictive nature of my life following the procedure, the probability of continued hospitalization and medical care, have been answered in a manner satisfactory to me.

9.   I recognize that following the implantation of the artificial heart, if successful, I will be dependent on an external life support system to

drive the artificial heart and that I will experience very limited mobility for the rest of my life with the artificial heart. No promises have been made to me about the extent of activity in which I will be able to engage after the surgery. I nevertheless accept limited mobility as one of the necessary results of the surgical procedure, and my continued life support with the artificial heart.

10. No representation has been made to me concerning the length of time I may be expected to live with my failing natural heart. There is no guarantee that the implantation of an artificial heart will add any additional time to my life expectancy. In fact this implantation might shorten my life.

11. I have discussed alternative treatments with my physician. These might include the possibility of no treatment, further drug treatment, attempts at possible surgical repair of my own failing heart and heart transplants. After having these alternatives and their probable effects on my case explained to me, I still authorize my physician to proceed with the implantation of an artificial heart device within my body.

12. I have been informed that in several medical centers cardiac assist pumps are under development. To the best of my physician's knowledge, none which will substantially improve my natural heart's function is presently available.

13. I recognize that following surgery I may require extended hospitalization and/or further treatment, including further surgery. I nevertheless assume the risk of such further hospitalization and treatment, including the financial cost thereof.

14. I hereby authorize the University of Utah Hospital, through its authorized agents, to dispose of or use for any purpose, any tissue or body parts which may be removed during the surgical procedures.

15. For the purpose of advancing medical knowledge, I authorize and consent to the admittance of medical students and other professional medical observers, in accordance with ordinary practices of the University of Utah Hospital, and to the use of video taping through closed circuit television, the taking of photographs (including motion pictures), the preparation of drawings and similar illustrative graphic material, and to the use of these graphic materials for scientific purposes. The U.S. Food and Drug Administration will have access to the data from this experiment. No public use of these materials will be made for purposes other than scientific presentation, and my rights to privacy and medical confidentiality will be maintained, except by explicit permission from me or my authorized representative.

16. I understand I am free at any time to withdraw my consent to participate in this experimental project, recognizing that the exercise of such an option after the artificial heart is in place may result in my death.

17. I have also reviewed with my physician and those with whom I live the considerable financial implications, including costs of surgery, hospitalization, continuing instrumentation, studies, monitoring and living with the artificial heart would impose upon me, and I am willing to accept these responsibilities. The University of Utah accepts no financial obligation for any harm or injury arising from this experiment. It is understood that none of the foregoing is intended to release my physicians, or the hospital, or their agents from liability for negligence.

18. I realize that by simply signing this form I do not obtain any rights to the artificial heart or its implantation. The following described circumstances justifying the failure to implant the total artificial heart are illustrative only and not all-inclusive. I understand that subsequent to my signing this form I could be deemed not acceptable for any reason whatsoever, including, but not limited to, death resulting from any cause or other medical complication (whether physiological, psychological, etc.).

I understand that Dr. DeVries or any other member of the artificial heart Evaluation Committee named below may determine at their sole discretion that implantation is not appropriate and the artificial heart will not be implanted.

(Name)	(Title)	(Position on Committee)
1. [CLAUDIA BERENSON	MD	PSYCHIATRIST]
2. [PEG MILLER		SOCIAL WORKER]
3. [HELEN KEE		DIRECTOR OF NURSING]
4. [FRED ANDERSON	MD	CARDIOLOGIST]
5. [THOMAS KEITH	MD	CARDIOLOGIST]
6. [ROSS WOOLLEY	PHD	IRB MONITOR]

I also realize that the available artificial heart may not be implanted if it is believed to be malfunctioning, if a crucial member of the surgical team is unavailable at the time surgery is scheduled, if my condition changes (for either the better or for the worse), or if additional complications are found during surgery. Within these limitations all decisions will be based on reasonable medical judgment.

___[W. DeVries]___ M.D.   ___[Barney Clark]___
(signature of physician   (patient's signature)
providing the above
information)

Dated this [29] day of [Nov] 19 [82]
at [8³⁰] o'clock [P] M.

_____   _____
              [L. D. Joyce]   [Grant W. Hauer]
                (witness)   (witness)

If - you - have - any - questions - regarding - this - experiment - you - may -
contact Dr. William DeVries at 581-5311.

I have signed the foregoing Special Consent at least 24 hours previously, and have had the opportunity to further consider the risks of the
procedure. After such additional consideration, it is still my desire to
have my physician proceed with the implantation of an artificial heart,
and I hereby confirm and ratify this Special consent.

_____ M.D.   _____
       [W. DeVries]   [Barney B. Clark]
   (signature of physician   (patient's signature)
      providing the above
         information)

Dated this [30] day of [Nov] 19 [82]
at [9⁵²] o'clock [P] M.

_____   _____
           [Chris C. Brown]   [Laurie Rowland]
                (witness)   (witness)

NOTE ADDED IN PROOF: A new and expanded version of the above
consent form has been approved by the IRB and FDA for the second implant patient. In addition to the disclosures and terms given above, the
new form includes (1) discussion of cardiac assist pumps, (2) the names
and relationships of two persons given power-of-attorney if the patient
is too sick or is incompetent to consent to further invasive procedures
or additional surgery, (3) a description of Dr. Barney Clark's experience
and cause of death, (4) the addition of complications suffered by Barney
Clark to the list given in the first consent form, (5) consent to autopsy
to remove the artificial heart, (6) recognition of intense media interest
and approval of use of written and audio-visual material by the media,
(7) expanded discussion of costs borne by third-party payors and the
university, and (8) the freedom to withdraw from experimental procedures while continuing to receive supportive care.—Ed.

Appendix B

PUBLICATIONS OF WILLIAM C. DEVRIES, M.D.

ARTICLES

Kwan-Gett, C. S., W. C. DeVries, and W. J. Kolff. "Performance of an Auto-regulatory Cardiac Prosthesis," *Circulation* (Supplement 3) 39 and 40 (1969): 111–128.

DeVries, W. C., C. S. Kwan-Gett, and W. J. Kolff. "Consumptive Coagulopathy, Shock and the Artificial Heart." *Trans Am Soc Artif Intern Organs* 16(1970): 29–36.

Kralios, A. C., C. S. Kwan-Gett, W. C. DeVries, and W. J. Kolff. "Transapical Left Ventricular Bypass" (Letters). *Appl Engineer Sci* 1(1973): 179–192.

DeVries, W. C., R. W. Anderson, W. G. Wolfe, and L. G. Alexander. "Pulmonary Capillary Filtration Following Oxygen Exposure." *Surg Forum* 24(1973): 224–226.

Alexander, L. G., W. C. DeVries, and R. W. Anderson. "Airway Pressure and Pulmonary Edema Formation." *Surg Forum* 24(1973): 231–234.

Wolfe, W. G., W. C. DeVries, R. W. Anderson, and D. C. Sabiston, Jr. "Changes in Pulmonary Capillary Filtration and Ventilatory Dead Space during Exposure to 95 Percent Oxygen." *J Surg Res* 16(1974): 312–317.

Duranceau, A., W. C. DeVries, W. G. Wolfe, and D. C. Sabiston, Jr. "Ventilatory Dead Space in Diagnosis of Acute Pulmonary Embolism." *Surg Forum* 25(1974): 229–231.

DeVries, W. C., and R. W. Anderson. "Physiologic and Pathologic Responses of the Pulmonary Circulation to High Flow Shunts," *Surg Forum* 26 (1975): 208–211.

Anderson, R. W., and W. C. DeVries. "Transvascular Fluid and Protein Dynamics in the Lung Following Hemorrhagic Shock." *J Surg Res* 20(1976): 281–290.

DeVries, W. C. "The Principles of Drainage of Wounds and Body Cavities." *OR Tech* 10(1978): 23–27.

DeVries, W. C., A. V. Seaber, and W. C. Seeley. "Unilateral Pulmonary Emphysema Created by Ligation of the Left Pulmonary Artery in Newborn Puppies." *Ann Thorac Surg* 27(1979): 154–160.

Crapo, R. O., A. H. Morris, S. L. Berlin, and W. C. DeVries. "Pulmonary Tissue Volume in Isolated Perfused Dog Lungs." *J Appl Physiol* 48(1980): 798–801.

McDonnell, M., A. C. Kralios, W. C. DeVries, F. L. Anderson, T. J. Tsagaris, and H. Kuida. "The Effect of the Pericardium on Ventricular Interaction in Brisket Disease." *Fed Proc* 39(1980): 1169.

Olsen, C. O., R. C. Hill, R. N. Jones, J. D. Sink, W. C. DeVries, and A. S. Wechsler. "Dimensional Analysis of Left Ventricular Systolic and Diastolic Properties in Man during Reperfusion Following Hypothermic Potassium Cardioplegia." *Surg Forum* 31(1980): 310–312.

Jarvik, R. K., T. R. Kessler, L. D. McGill, D. B. Olsen, W. C. DeVries, J. Deneris, J. T. Blaylock, and W. J. Kolff. "Determinants of Pannus Formation in Long-surviving Artificial Heart Calves, and Its Prevention." *Trans Am Soc Artif Intern Organs* 27(1981): 90–93.

Olsen, D. B., W. C. DeVries, P. E. Oyer, B. A. Reitz, J. Murashita, W. J. Kolff, N. Daitch, R. K. Jarvik, and R. Gaykowski. "Artificial Heart Implantation, Later Cardiac Transplantation in the Calf." *Trans Am Soc Artif Intern Organs* 27(1981): 132–136.

Olsen, D. B., W. C. DeVries, J. Murashita, P. Oyer, B. Reitz, R. Blaylock, R. Gaykowski, and W. J. Kolff. "Long-term Total Body Preservation While Awaiting a Suitable Cardiac Donor." *J Artif Organs* 5(1981): 53.

Olsen, D. B., W. C. DeVries, W. J. Kolff, O. H. Frazier, and S. H. Rahimtoola. "Indeterminate Circulatory Support with the Artificial Heart." *Trans Am Soc Artif Intern Organs* 28(1982): 652–655.

Smith, D. L., W. L. Hastings, L. D. Joyce, and W. C. DeVries. "Case Report: Cardiopulmonary Bypass during Implantation of the Permanent Total Artificial Heart." *Proceedings of the American Academy of Cardiovascular Perfusion* 4(1983): 181–185.

DeVries, W. C., and L. D. Joyce. "The Artificial Heart." *Ciba Clinical Symposia* 35(1983): 32 pp.

Morton, W. A., W. C. DeVries, W. H. Dobelle, K. D. Serkes, R. Sheridan, and D. Dennis. "Impact of Regulations on Artificial Organs Research." *Trans Am Soc Artif Intern Organs* 29(1983): 770–773.

DeVries, W. C., L. D. Joyce, W. L. Hastings, D. B. Olsen, R. K. Jarvik, and W. J. Kolff. "The Permanent Clinical Implantation of the Utah Total Artificial Heart." (Abstract). *Am Soc Artif Intern Organs Abstracts* 12(1983): 2.

Taylor, A., Jr., P. E. Christian, W. C. DeVries, F. L. Datz, and L. D. Joyce. "Gated Radionuclide Studies of the Artificial Heart in Vivo: Case Report." *Noninvas Med Imag* 1(1984): 3–7.

DeVries, W. C., J. L. Anderson, L. D. Joyce, F. L. Anderson, E. H. Hammond, R. K. Jarvik, and W. J. Kolff. "Clinical Use of the Total Artificial Heart," *N Engl J Med* 310(1984): 273–278.

Raymond, J. L., W. C. DeVries, and L. D. Joyce. "Nutrition's Role in the First Total Artificial Heart Patient: Implications for Future Patients," *Am Diet Assoc* 84(1984): 532–535.

Hastings, W. L., L. D. Joyce, W. C. DeVries, P. B. Olsen, S. D. Nielsen, and

W. J. Kolff. "Drive System Management in the Clinical Implantation of the Jarvik-7 Total Artificial Heart," *Trans Int Soc Artif Organs* (in press).

Pace, N. L., M. M. Matthews, T. H. Stanley, W. C. DeVries, and L. D. Joyce. "Anesthetic Management of the First Permanent Orthotopic, Prosthetic Cardiac Replacement (Total Artificial Heart) in Man." *Anesthesia and Analgesia* 63 (in press).

DeVries, W. C., et al. "Clinical Use of the Total Artifical Heart" (Abstract). *International Synopses* (in press).

DeVries, W. C., and L. D. Joyce. "The Implantation of the Total Artificial Heart for the Treatment of Endstage Cardiomyopathy." *J Thorac Surg* (in press).

BOOK CHAPTERS

Moody, F. G., and W. C. DeVries. "The Esophagus and Diaphragmatic Hernias." In *Hardy's Textbook of Surgery*, edited by J. D. Hardy, pp. 469–496. Philadelphia: J. P. Lippincott, 1982.

DeVries, W. C. "The Total Artificial Heart," In *Gibbon's Surgery of the Chest*, edited by D. C. Sabiston and J. C. Spencer, pp. 1629–1636. Philadelphia: W. B. Saunders, 1983.

PAPERS READ AT MEETINGS

Olsen, D. B., P. Oyer, B. Reitz, W. C. DeVries, J. Kolff, J. Murashita, R. Blaylock, and R. Gaykowski. "Cardiac Transplantation in Twin Calves." Paper presented at the annual meeting of the American College of Veterinary Surgeons, New Orleans, 1981.

Christian, P. E., W. L. Hastings, W. C. DeVries, F. L. Datz, and A. T. Taylor. "Multigated Radionuclide Studies of the Artificial Heart." Paper presented at the Western Regional Conference of the Society of Nuclear Medicine, San Diego, California, 1982.

Olsen, D. B., W. C. DeVries, L. D. Joyce, K. D. Murray, Y. Hamanaka, B. Chiang, and W. J. Kolff. "Cardiac Transplantation in Calves Following Prolonged Maintenance on the Total Artificial Heart." Paper presented at the annual meeting of the Samson Thoracic Surgery Society, Colorado Springs, Colorado, 1983.

Armstrong, J. D., W. C. DeVries, L. D. Joyce, and F. L. Anderson. "The Implanted Total Artificial Heart: Imaging Perspectives." Paper presented at the annual meeting of the Association of University Radiologists, Mobile, Alabama, 1983.

Smith, D. L., W. L. Hastings, L. D. Joyce, and W. C. DeVries. "Case Report: Cardiopulmonary Bypass during Implantation of Permanent Total Artificial Heart." Paper presented at the annual meeting of the American Academy of Cardiac Perfusion, San Diego, California, 1983.

Contributors

LAWRENCE K. ALTMAN is medical correspondent and writer of "The Doctor's World" for the *New York Times*. He is also clinical associate professor of medicine at New York University Medical School and a member of the Institute of Medicine of the National Academy of Sciences. Dr. Altman received his A.B. in government from Harvard and his M.D. from Tufts University. He is a fellow of the American College of Physicians and the American College of Epidemiology. He received the Blakeslee Award from the American Heart Association for his coverage of the artificial heart story.

DAVID BLUMENTHAL is executive director of the Center for Health Policy and Management and lecturer in public policy at the John F. Kennedy School of Government, Harvard University. He is also on the staff of Massachusetts General Hospital. Dr. Blumenthal received his M.D. from Harvard and his master's degree in public policy from the John F. Kennedy School of Government. From 1977 to 1979 he was a professional staff member of the Senate Subcommittee on Health and Scientific Research, chaired by Senator Edward Kennedy, and drafted legislation regarding health care technology, health maintenance organizations, and preventive health services. His research interests include the nature and consequences of university-industry relationships, the influence of ownership on health care organizations, and the development of federal policy toward health care technology.

JOHN A. BOSSO is associate professor of clinical pharmacy and adjunct associate professor of pediatrics at the University of Utah College of Pharmacy and School of Medicine. He received his B.S. and Pharm. D. degrees from the State University of New York at Buffalo. His research areas include evaluating the efficacy and pharmacokinetics of anti-infective agents. He is chairman of the University of Utah Institutional Review Board for Research with Human Subjects.

ALEXANDER MORGAN CAPRON is professor of law, ethics, and public policy at Georgetown University, Washington, D.C., where he specializes in the social and legal aspects of medicine and science. He received his B.A. from Swarthmore and his LL.B. from Yale, where he was an officer of the *Yale Law Journal*. He is a fellow and board member of the Institute of Society,

Ethics and the Life Sciences; a member of the Institute of Medicine; and a board member of the American Society of Law and Medicine. From 1979 to 1983 he served as the executive director of the President's Commission for the Study of Ethical Problems in Medicine and Biomedical and Behavioral Research, work recognized by the American College of Physicians with the 1984 Rosenthal Foundation Award. He is a frequent contributor to professional journals and has written several books, including *Catastrophic Diseases: Who Decides What?* (with Jay Katz) and *Law, Science, and Medicine* (with J. Areen, P. King, and S. Goldberg).

C. THOMAS CASKEY is professor of medicine and director of the R. J. Kleberg Center for Human Genetics at Baylor College of Medicine in Houston. He is a Howard Hughes Medical Investigator. He received his M.D. from Duke University, where he received the Borden Research Award as a medical student and was a Josiah Macy, Jr., Faculty Scholar. Dr. Caskey is chairman of the Mammalian Genetics Study Section of the National Institutes of Health and of the Biochemistry Test Committee of the National Board of Medical Examiners. He is a member of the American Society for Clinical Investigation and has served on the editorial boards of *Archives of Biochemistry and Biophysics, Annals of Internal Medicine,* and the *Journal of Biological Chemistry.* His research interests are in clinical and molecular genetics.

ERIC J. CASSELL is clinical professor of public health, Cornell University Medical College, and director of the Cornell Program for the Study of Ethics and Values in Medicine. He received his B.S. from Queens College, New York; his M.A. from Columbia; and his M.D. from New York University School of Medicine. He is a diplomate, American Board of Internal Medicine; fellow, Institute of Society, Ethics and the Life Sciences; and a member of the Institute of Medicine. He has published more than one hundred articles in scientific journals and is the author of *The Healer's Art: A New Perspective on the Doctor-Patient Relationship* and *Talking with Patients: Theory and Practice in Doctor-Patient Communication.*

WILLIAM A. CHECK is a free-lance medical and science journalist. He has a Ph.D. in microbiology from Case Western Reserve University and has done postdoctoral research on herpes viruses at the University of Chicago. Dr. Check was an associate editor for *JAMA Medical News* for three years, and he continues to write for *JAMA* as well as other medical and scientific publications and lay magazines.

RENÉE C. FOX is the Annenberg Professor of the Social Sciences at the University of Pennsylvania, where she has joint professorial appointments in the Departments of Sociology, Psychiatry, and Medicine and in the School of Nursing. Dr. Fox has a Ph.D. in sociology from Radcliffe College/Harvard University and holds honorary degrees from the University of Pennsylvania, the Medical College of Pennsylvania, St. Joseph's University in Philadelphia, Smith College, and Katholieke Universiteit Leuven in Belgium. Her major teaching and research interests—sociology of medicine, medical science and technology, medical education, and medical ethics—have involved her in first-hand studies in the United States, Europe (chiefly Belgium), Central Africa (principally Zaire), and recently in the People's Republic of China. She has served as a member of the board of directors of the American Association for the Advancement of Science (1977–1981), of the Council of the Institute of Medicine (1979–1982), and as a member of the President's Commission for the Study of Ethical Problems in Medicine and Biomedical and Behavioral Research (1979–1981). She is the author of *Experiment Perilous: Physicians and Patients Facing the Unknown;* coauthor (with Willy De Craemer) of *The Emerging Physician: A Sociological Approach to the Development of a Congolese Medical Profession;* coauthor (with Judith P. Swazey) of *The Courage to Fail: A Social View of Organ Transplants and Dialysis;* and author of *Essays in Medical Sociology: Journeys into the Field.*

DENISE GRADY is a free-lance writer and a contributor to *Discover* magazine, where she spent three years as a staff writer. She has written several stories on the artificial heart, the first one in 1981. She has also been a senior editor of *Medical Month* magazine and an assistant editor of the *New England Journal of Medicine* and *Physics Today* magazine. She has received journalism awards from the National High Blood Pressure Education Program and the Squibb Corporation, the National Society of Professional Engineers, and the National Council for Geographic Education. She holds a bachelor's degree in biology from the State University of New York at Stony Brook and a master's in English from the University of New Hampshire.

ALBERT R. JONSEN is professor of ethics in medicine and chief, Division of Medical Ethics in the Department of Medicine, School of Medicine, University of California, San Francisco. He has a Ph.D. from Yale. He has served on the National Commission for the Protection of Human Subjects of Biomedical and Behavioral Research (1974–1978) and the President's Commission for the Study of Ethical Problems in Medicine and Biomedical and Behavioral Research (1979–1982). He is a member of the Institute of Medicine; a fellow of the Institute of Society, Ethics and the Life Sciences; and a board member of the American Society of Law and Medicine. He is an author (with M. Seigler and W. Winslade) of *Clinical Ethics.*

JAY KATZ is John A. Garver Professor of Law and Psychoanalysis at Yale Law School. He received his M.D. from Harvard. He is a member of the Institute of Medicine and on the editorial board of several journals pertaining to law, psychiatry, and ethics. He received the Isaac Ray award from the American Psychiatric Association and the William C. Menninger award from the American College of Physicians. He is author of *Experimentation with Human Beings* and coauthor (with Alexander Morgan Capron) of *Catastrophic Diseases: Who Decides What?* His most recent book, *The Silent World of Doctor and Patient*, was published in 1984.

GILBERT S. OMENN is professor of medicine and of environmental health and dean of the School of Public Health and Community Medicine at the University of Washington, Seattle. He received his A.B. from Princeton, his

M.D. from Harvard, and a Ph.D. in genetics from the University of Washington. His research and public policy interests lie in areas of genetic predisposition to environmental and occupational health hazards, the improvement of science-based risk analysis, and applications of genetic engineering. From 1977 to 1981, Dr. Omenn served as a deputy to Frank Press, President Carter's science and technology advisor and director of the White House Office of Science and Technology Policy, and then as associate director for human resources in the Office of Management and Budget. He has been a visiting fellow at the Brookings Institution and Princeton University. He is coauthor (with L. Lave) of *Clearing the Air: Reforming the Clean Air Act* and coeditor (with A. Hollaender) of *Genetic Control of Environmental Pollutants.*

CHASE N. PETERSON is president of the University of Utah. His M.D. is from Harvard University, and he completed an internship, residency, and fellowship at Yale University. He was university coordinator for the Artificial Heart Project and held the position of vice president for health sciences when the first artificial heart was implanted at the University of Utah Medical Center. He has worked on studies of radioactive fallout in southern Utah, Universal National Service for the Ford Foundation, and chaired a conference on the health effects of nuclear war.

STANLEY JOEL REISER is director and professor of Humanities and Technology in Health Care at The University of Texas Health Science Center at Houston. He received his A.B. at Columbia College; M.D. at State University of New York, Downstate Medical Center; M.P.A. at Harvard, John F. Kennedy School of Government; and Ph.D. in the history of medicine at Harvard. He was formerly associate professor and director, Program in History of Medicine, Harvard Medical School. He is author of *Medicine and the Reign of Technology* and coeditor of *Ethics in Medicine: Historical Perspectives and Contemporary Concerns* and of *The Machine at the Bedside: Strategies for Using Technology in Patient Care.*

JOANN ELLISON RODGERS, deputy director, Office of Public Affairs, The Johns Hopkins Medical Institution, was a science writer for Hearst newspapers for eighteen years and remains a frequent contributor to many science, women's, and family magazines. She received her M.S. from Columbia University Graduate School of Journalism. She is immediate past-president of the National Association of Science Writers, a director of the Council for the Advancement of Science Writing, an instructor in the Department of Epidemiology at Johns Hopkins University School of Hygiene and Public Health, and a frequent lecturer on science communication. She has received awards for her work from the Lasker Foundation, the American Heart Association, the American Cancer Society, the National Council for Medical Research, and the Cystic Fibrosis Foundation.

MARGERY W. SHAW is director of the Institute for the Interprofessional Study of Health Law and professor of medical genetics at The University of Texas Health Science Center at Houston. Dr. Shaw received her M.D. from the

University of Michigan, her J.D. from the University of Houston, and an honorary D.Sc. from the University of Evansville. She is Andrew D. White Professor-at-Large at Cornell University and past president of the American Society of Human Genetics and the Genetics Society of America. She is a fellow of the American College of Legal Medicine, on the board of directors of the American Society of Law and Medicine, and served on the Director's Advisory Committee of the National Institutes of Health. Dr. Shaw has been a visiting professor at Yale University, the University of North Carolina, and the University of Utah.

RICHARD J. ZECKHAUSER is professor of political economy, John F. Kennedy School of Government, Harvard University. He holds a Ph.D. in economics from Harvard. He is coauthor of *A Primer for Policy Analysis*, of *Demographic Dimensions of the New Republic*, and editor of *What Role for Government?* His research, which has resulted in more than seventy published articles, is divided between conceptual work in economics and assessments of policy issues. His work in health has addressed the valuation of life, catastrophic health insurance, patient heterogeneity, the allocation of resources to biomedical research, and the regulation of various aspects of the health care system.

Index